Life

AFTER LUPUS

What's Your Autoimmune Name?

ANDREA LENDE

ISBN 978-1-0980-3334-7 (paperback)
ISBN 978-1-0980-3335-4 (digital)

Christian Faith Publishing, Inc.
832 Park Avenue
Meadville, PA 16335
www.christianfaithpublishing.com

Printed in the United States of America

Contents

Life Before Lupus

The phrase "chasing dreams" sums up my early adult years. It seemed I was always chasing a dream.

At first I chased college and completed a bachelor's degree with two majors and a minor at a private Lutheran college in Minnesota. Mid-completion, I took a break for about two years and chased business. Eventually I returned to college to finish my education. I majored in psychology and business administration with a minor in Latin. As I finished college, I found it was difficult to find employment in the community so moved to Minneapolis to accept a position with the government.

When I was twenty-five, my husband and I discovered the joy of flying. From the very first takeoff in a very small Cessna, I was completely starstruck. I immediately fell in love with flying. Every takeoff was magnificent, and as the earth beneath me disappeared, the most beautiful patchwork quilt appeared. It was breathtaking. I began to see the miracle of this earth and appreciated the Maker of this great world in a whole new way.

I so enjoyed takeoffs and landings at sunrise and sunset. I sought out those times to fly because they were the most beautiful. In North Dakota, one could see for miles. Once in the air, the earth, the world, and the troubles we encounter seemed to disappear. The sensation and freedom of leaving them behind was always present. The calm of the morning and evening were very desirable flying times for me because of the comfort they provided as well as the beauty of the rising and setting of the sun. Once the sun came up, the winds started. We were accustomed to twenty- to thirty-knot winds on any given day. So, it was far more desirable to fly early or later to avoid the gusty wind conditions that always made for tricky takeoffs and landings.

A few years after we started flying, we moved to Minneapolis, Minnesota, where we continued flight lessons at a flight school in St. Paul, Minnesota. On one occasion, I was flying with an FAA pilot, and he set up an adventure into the Minneapolis-St. Paul International Airport. We were flying a Cessna 150 into the Minneapolis-St. Paul International Airport where we landed and then taxied and took off again. We were situated between huge jets, and even though they were so much bigger than we were, I could still see the pilots through the cockpit windows. The pilot I was flying with calmed my nerves and told me that they were probably looking at us with envy wishing they were flying a small plane again. One never gets over the feeling of trolling around in a small airplane at low speeds.

I was challenged with flight test after flight test during those early flying days. There were both written tests and in-flight tests for every new rating. Almost all of my competitors were young men. There were very few women taking flight lessons thirty years ago. And I wanted to beat all the guys. So, I pushed and pushed at every lesson and every book I read in order to pass each test with professionalism and pride.

Winter flying was challenging because it was so cold in the upper midwest. The below freezing and subzero temperatures were brutal. Some days it was too cold to fly because of possible engine trouble, so we stayed on the ground and studied.

I was working full-time along with flying part-time, and attending ground school classes in the evening, eventually earning a professional pilot degree from a local college that provided ground school courses. Since I had already received a bachelor's degree, all the rest of my classes transferred to earn the PPD.

There were many nights that I didn't get home until after 9:00 p.m. and started work early at 7:00 a.m. in order to allow time after work to fly. This fast-paced, high-thrill, adrenalin rush time took its toll on my body. I also was not taking care of me as I should have been. I was eating on the run, so it was fast-food or no food. And by the time I came home, I'd be found eating a bowl of cereal before bedtime. Ignoring my health led to significant health problems that took years for me to reverse.

As someone who had already chased a number of dreams, I had told my husband that flying was the last dream I would chase. If I didn't make a dollar by the time I was thirty, I was done chasing. I became a flight instructor by the time I was twenty-nine, so I had surpassed my goal. However, the damage to my body had already been done. And one day, my body just broke.

During the months and years of healing that followed, my eyes never stopped looking skyward. I was always spotting air traffic sometimes more so than traffic on the road. One day as I was driving, I looked skyward, and with tears in my eyes, I told God that although flying was my passion, I knew His plan was better, and I would wait to see what He had in store for me. I had no idea that the adventures ahead would be to save my life as He was saving my soul.

Solo Journey

It seems that some of the most difficult journeys we face in life are also the times we experience the most growth. And many times, these most difficult journeys are solo journeys.

Most of us have an all-important journey that we will embark upon on our own. We will be ministered to by the Holy Spirit. We may be fortunate enough to come into God's presence. Jesus will certainly intercede on our behalf. And all of these wonderful spiritual gifts will be experienced with awe and wonder. They will carry us through some of the most difficult days we will experience on this earth.

When we enter the miraculous, there are few people close to us who will be able to handle the difficulties we will face. Our friends will scatter. Our families will distance themselves, and rightly so. They haven't been given God's mercy and grace and strength for our journey—only we have.

My husband walked this difficult journey from illness to health with me. He watched me waste away to almost nothing and then regain my strength little by little until I was well again. I am thankful for his constant strength that I was able to rely on during that season. I am also thankful for the journey that lay ahead of me way back then and is now in my rearview mirror.

May God be with you and your journey in a way that is so miraculous as to change your life and the lives of those around you.

Leaving Paradise

My husband and I loved vacationing in Hawaii. We had found Hawaii to be our little bit of heaven on earth. This was partly because we grew up in the north part of the country where the winter temperatures were often below zero for days on end and summer lasted about two months. The snow never left the ground once it came sometime in October. We had the benefit of escaping from time to time because in our early twenties we became an airline couple. Our first trip to Hawaii was quite by accident. We hopped on a flight to Denver and would decide where our next stop was going to be once we were up in the air. After a few more flights, we found ourselves in the most beautiful place we had ever been. There were the most aromatic smells of island flowers, tropical breezes that soothed the skin, and sun that touched our skin and warmed us through and through. Hawaii would become our very favorite place to take time and rest from our busy lives.

After a number of trips to the beautiful islands of Hawaii, we were headed home yet one more time. We had enjoyed the warm sandy beaches, lazy days, and lovely accommodations. The ambiance of the hotel alone is worth the flight from the mainland to the islands. It is so festive and yet quiet and relaxing with tropical breezes gently blowing through the atrium and lobby. I have always felt those breezes as being healing to my body, mind, and spirit. Every time we walked through the door of the hotel, the staff greeted us wearing Hawaiian leis made from their breathtaking island flowers that smelled like a bouquet of the most fragrant flowers I have ever had the pleasure of smelling. It is truly the stuff that perfumes are made of. As we prepared to leave this little bit of heaven on earth, we had no idea that this would be our last day on their beautiful island for a long time to come.

The morning of our departure, I stole just thirty more minutes soaking up the warm sun and breathing in the balmy salty air poolside. Because I was already dressed for breakfast, I hadn't put any sunscreen on and had no idea that this one action would set the course for the next three years of my life. Lupus is exacerbated with the sun's rays, but I didn't know that at the time. The result of the warm sun and all its rays would result in the beginning of a long battle for my health and my life.

We ate a lovely breakfast after those few precious moments stolen in the sun and proceeded to the airport for a very long journey home. As an airline couple, we flew standby on all of our flights, so we waited patiently at the gate for the first segment of our trip from Kauai to Honolulu. As we took off that beautiful morning, I found myself gasping for air. I couldn't get a full breath in or out. I started to panic but attempted to slow my breathing down as much as I could until we landed. As we got off the first flight to start the next segment back to the mainland, I told my husband that I needed to see a doctor at the airport before boarding the next plane. I wasn't even sure that there was a physician at the airport, but we did find the location of a medical office on site and walked as quickly as we could to the office. There were no other patients waiting, so we were quickly escorted to the doctor's office. He listened to my airways and said that I was moving air in and out well. He didn't know what was causing the sensation that I was experiencing, but his words were affirming enough that we decided to continue on with our journey.

On the next five-hour flight to Los Angeles, I was, again, unable to breathe easily. I took antihistamines to help keep my airways open and thankfully dozed in and out of sleep throughout the flight. However, as I fell in and out of consciousness, I felt as though I was under water unable to maintain the very basic function—breathing. I had to concentrate on every breath I took to complete it. I had to start regulating a process that we don't even think about regulating at any given moment in time. We take for granted that our breath will be given to us without thinking about it. We don't ask our heart to beat or our blood to pump or our lungs to expand and give us the capability to take in oxygen. But at this point in time, I had to consciously think about how to breathe in and out and how to slow it down when it didn't seem to be a complete breath.

Our flight landed in Los Angeles, and as we waited for the next flight to Colorado, the symptoms continued. Thankfully, we were denied seats on our last segment because there were none to be had. I was very thankful that we didn't have to get on another plane. I simply didn't see how I could withstand another few hours of the laborious breathing I had been going through all the while locked into a confined space such as the tube of an airplane.

We stayed in a hotel until the next day, and I took more antihistamines hoping that my airways would stay open and the struggle to take a breath would be eased. The ease of breathing didn't return through the night; however, I was so exhausted from this new physical difficulty that sleep finally took over. Thankfully, I rested on and off throughout the night, so the remaining three-hour trip was tolerable. We made it home not knowing that the next three years would hold a long, painful journey from sickness to health.

First Round of Doctors

The symptoms that I had experienced on the way back from Hawaii had seemed to become less severe over the next few days, and I dismissed the idea of anything being seriously wrong for a short time. However, one day at work just after finishing up lunch, I was, again, under the spell of laborious breathing. This time, I immediately scheduled an appointment with my doctor and left work early to embark on a health journey that would be one of the most difficult journeys of my life.

My primary care physician didn't really know what was affecting my breathing issues and recommended I see an allergist. I asked if there was any possibility of getting into one that afternoon because I really didn't want to go home with the same sensation of not being able to breathe any longer. She made a few phone calls and scheduled me with an allergist who was the first of many doctors I would see over the next few years.

The allergist took a look at me and listened to my symptoms and asked me at least one hundred questions. The questions didn't seem to have any cohesiveness to them or relevance to my condition. I couldn't tell what he was looking to discover because they all seemed so random and didn't lead to any definitive diagnosis that he spoke of during the visit. However, he knew exactly what he was looking for and ordered so many blood tests that I thought the phlebotomist was going to use every vial in her box. The tests he ordered were specialized tests that had to be sent out of state for diagnostic purposes, so we would wait several weeks for the results. The doctor didn't tell me what he was testing for, and at that time, I hadn't asked him what he thought might be the problem. I just answered his questions and gave lots and lots of blood to be tested.

I left the allergist's office with no information about a possible diagnosis but seemed satisfied that someone was looking into what was causing the inability for me to take a full breath. I continued on the only regimen I knew—taking antihistamines to keep my airways open. This resulted in constant extreme drowsiness and fatigue. The fatigue I was now experiencing coupled with difficulty in breathing would become my new normal for years to come.

Over the next coming days and nights, my breathing became laborious again, and I contacted the allergist. He recommended staying calm when I was frantic as my symptoms worsened and my desire to check into the emergency room was overwhelming. At one point, he advised me to go if I really felt that I needed the assistance. I did go, and the emergency room doctor recommended I see a doctor who could test me for gall bladder problems because he was suspicious that this could be causing the stomach distress that was affecting my breathing. The appointment was scheduled, and yet another doctor came into our world to try and assess my condition. Before I left the emergency room, the doctor looked intently at me and said that I seemed to be a stressed out young lady. At that time, I simply thought that the illness was the stressor, but I would later discover that I needed to alter my way of life and address my emotional and spiritual needs to become completely well.

Gall Bladder

The gall bladder doctor examined me and decided it was worthy to order a test to determine if my stomach distress was, indeed, due to gall bladder issues. I had to take some extremely large pills prior to the X-ray in order to complete the test. These pills would dissolve and the matter distributed throughout my body so they could take whatever X-ray's they needed to of the gall bladder and determine if the gall bladder needed to be removed. I explained to him that I was allergic to so many things and that I was likely going to have an allergic reaction to the pills that were prescribed for me. So, he suggested coming to the emergency room to take them just in case a reaction occurred, and they would treat me immediately. We scheduled the date and time to come to the emergency room and ingest the pills so that it coincided with the appointment scheduled for the X-ray's needed.

On the appointed day and time, my husband and I went into the emergency room, and I started taking the pills. Within about fifteen minutes, I felt that my airways were closing and was immediately brought into a room where the staff started the usual medications for such a reaction. They put an IV in with an assortment of Benadryl, Tagamet, and other standard medications for allergic reactions. The Benadryl shot in the IV was memorable because it caused a reaction that left me unable to breathe for a short period. In fact, I couldn't breathe at all or speak to alert anyone. The sensation was that of drowning. With a terrified look in my eyes, I was trying to grab my husband's arm but couldn't reach him to alert him that something was very wrong. When I could finally talk and breathe,

the nurse explained to me that sometimes that happens when the shot is admitted too quickly. That was a sensation that I never wanted to experience again, and haven't to this day.

After a few more moments, another very strange sensation started. The room started spinning. The doctor was called in immediately. He asked me if the room was spinning left or right. I told him the direction, and he stated, "That cannot be because that would be indicative of heart problems." I asked him what was in the IV drip, and he stated that Tagamet was one of the medications. I quickly told him that I was allergic to it and to stop that medication in the IV drip. He didn't seem to want to believe me, but they stopped the Tagamet and the spinning slowed down and eventually was gone. However, the effects of the drugs administered that evening affected me for the next couple of days.

The next morning my husband was going to be gone for work, and as I awoke, I knew something was terribly wrong. Half of my lower body was kind of numb, giving the sensation of pins and needles in them. It felt like the lower half of my body was asleep. As I lay in bed, the situation worsened. I placed a call to the doctor who said that it was probably a result of the medications I was given the day before and if the sensation continued to worsen that I should go to the hospital. Of course over the next hour or so, the pins and needles and numbness seemed to be creeping up my torso. I did not want to go to the hospital because every time I did, I ended up worse than I was before being admitted. So, I called a friend and asked if she would mind if I spent the day with her family just in case I needed someone to drive me to the hospital later that day. Fortunately, after the symptoms initially worsened, they started to subside by evening, and I was able to drive home fairly comfortably.

I had only one more appointment with the gall bladder doctor. When I went to the appointment, he wasn't much interested in pursuing more tests and began a series of questions about the physicians I had recently seen. When I told him I had really only seen my primary care physician and an allergist, he asked me what the allergist was testing me for with all the blood I'd given. I told him I wasn't sure, and we called him from his office. In speaking with the allergist, he said that he had interned at a lupus clinic during his training, and he suspected that that's what I was dealing with so was testing my blood work accordingly. However, the results would take about three weeks to come back because there were only a few places in the country that could do the appropriate tests. I got pretty emotional at that point because I knew that something seriously life-changing could be in front of me with no warning that my body would not be functioning as it should. The gall bladder doctor was very sweet and sympathetic. I remember he hugged me for a moment and then suggested that we wait until the tests came back before he and I scheduled anything further. That was the last time I saw him.

My Ally

Simultaneous to my symptoms starting, my cousin was diagnosed with lupus. Her mother, my aunt, would become one of my closest allies. We talked every day for months. We went over every symptom and compared my symptoms to my cousin's symptoms. All were so similar. The fatigue was overwhelming. More symptoms would follow. I would suffer from dry mouth and dry eyes, aches and pains in my joints, weird skin rashes, cold extremities, continued intestinal issues, and the list grew. I'm not sure how I made it to work every day, but I continued to work as I dealt with all the medical problems that I was experiencing and would soon encounter. I read and studied everything I could on various illnesses, and my aunt would do the same. And we compared our copious notes every day. My aunt was truly my strength during those times.

Most autoimmune diseases take years to diagnose with so many misdiagnoses that we are deemed hypochondriacs in many cases. I was thankful that the allergist knew exactly what tests to take because he had interned in a lupus clinic and proceeded to take the tests necessary to know what I might be dealing with at the onset of most of my symptoms. The tests came back with elevated ANA (antinuclear antibodies), so we knew an autoimmune disease was more than likely on its way. There are so many autoimmune diseases that had horrible symptoms and prognoses that I wasn't sure which one to hope for. It took over a year to determine which one it would be.

Gastroenterologist

The intestinal problems I suffered with were almost insur-
mountable. I finally discovered that the breathing problems weren't
a result of lung issues but of intestinal distress. My stomach was in
such distress that I couldn't move my abdomen in and out to get a
full breath. So many medications were prescribed, but to no avail. I
was allergic to most of them. I started seeing a gastroenterologist, and
he completed every *-opsy* that could be done. We actually completed
an endoscopy without any medications during the procedure because
of all the allergies I had to medications.

The first of many tests was the endoscopy. Generally this procedure requires a medication to deaden the gag reflex; however, we
didn't use that, so the gag reflex was in full effect. Another medication that is typically administered is one that almost puts you to
sleep. We didn't use that either. The gastroenterologist was a doctor
from Germany who had done the procedure in the past without any
medications, and he informed the nurse that we would be doing the
same for my procedure. She had never seen this done before. After
the test was completed, she said that she never wanted to do this
procedure without medications again.

The date and time was set for the procedure, and I drove myself
to the medical facility ready to deal with whatever was in front of
me for the next hour or so. I was greeted and asked to fill out forms,
change into a gown, and wait until the doctor was available and
ready. When it was my turn for the procedure, I was asked to lie on a
very short cold metal table. He explained how everything was going
to go and that he would be talking me through the procedure step

by step as it was happening. He was going to insert a hose down my throat and into my stomach. He said that it would feel like I couldn't breathe but that I would be able to breathe through my nose. So, I was to remain as calm as possible in order for him to do all the things he needed to do in order to complete the test.

The doctor was ready to begin and picked up a device from a nearby table, which kind of looked like the modern-day handheld controller kids use to play video games. He told me that he was going to complete all the necessary manipulations through this device once the tube was inserted down my throat. The first time he attempted to insert the large circular tube down my throat, my body reacted fairly violently, and he almost dropped the handheld device. He told me that I had to remain calm because the device that I almost caused him to drop cost tens of thousands of dollars, and we didn't want him to drop or break it. He put the tube down my throat once again, and he talked me through the procedure step by step. Every once in a while the gag reflex would take over, and I would have to calm it down in order for him to proceed. He completed the procedure and removed the tube from my throat. The nurse was rather distressed about how the procedure went; however, I felt quite accomplished at having gone through it without any of the standard medications. And I was happy to leave the hospital without having to stay in recovery like the rest of the people I was surrounded by in the recovery room. I left fifteen minutes later and drove myself to work.

It is extremely difficult to identify intestinal issues, and after the heroic measures we took to complete the tests I underwent, there was no diagnosis. So, the search continued. A few of my friends recommended a naturopathic physician because they had taken a more natural approach to their health with favorable results. I went to see a naturopathic doctor that was recommended, and the long path toward healing began.

The Journey Toward Healing

The first appointment I had with the naturopathic physician was full of questions by the doctor and a long questionnaire that had to be filled out. He seemed to want to know every minute detail of my life, my health, and my body. After an extremely long interchange, he advised a week of no solid food. He prescribed a powder that turned into a liquid meal replacement packed with the highest quality nutrition that would ultimately sustain me for the next ninety days. I took on the challenge because I was desperate for anything that would alleviate the tremendous stomach pain I was suffering with.

Day by day, my stomach pain eased a bit, and by the end of the week, I was enjoying the benefit of lessened pain so much that I didn't want to start eating food. I called the doctor and asked him for his recommendation. His response was unlike any other that I had received from previous doctors. He told me that I was blessed to feel no need to start eating right away and to continue on the liquid meal replacement until he could see me again. Because my health was in such jeopardy, we had frequent appointments, which typically went the same way. He would ask me questions, make recommendations, and tell me to stay on the liquid meal replacement.

On one of the early appointments I had with the naturopathic doctor, another fairly nontraditional recommendation was made. He recommended that I do enemas one to two times a day to help alleviate continued stomach pain and frequent bladder infections. His nurse said that they recommend this procedure for a lot of cancer patients as well and that they can be safely conducted for up to three years. There were days that it took three enemas in order to alleviate the severe stomach pain and allow me to breathe better. I tucked away the three-year time frame in my mind even though I didn't know at that time that this procedure too would become my new normal for the next three years.

Soon I started purchasing the liquid meal replacement at the warehouse because I was going through so much of it that it was more cost effective to buy in bulk, and the naturopathic doctor couldn't keep enough of it in stock to meet my needs. The cost was just over $60 a canister, and I went through one every three days. We were spending a lot for my sustenance, but it was necessary for my healing. I had lost about forty pounds by that time and was thankful then that I had the extra pounds to lose.

Perfect Meet

After about ninety days of seeing the naturopathic doctor, I met a woman at the warehouse when I was buying the liquid meal replacement. This meet would change the path I would find for complete and total healing.

On one particular day, there was a woman I had not previously met at the warehouse. She asked me how I liked the drink. I told her I absolutely loved it and that it had saved my life. She asked me how I liked the taste to which I, again, replied that *I loved it*! She said that there were others who didn't feel that way and had complained about the taste. The revelation that came to me then was that God had blessed me with the grace to love this drink as He required it for my healing.

This same woman had started telling me about her son who had been sick after I shared my health story with her. She said that her son had become so ill that she had almost lost him. He was a young boy at that time, and she used organic foods to nurse him back to health. He had to learn to eat all over again, and she started with very simple steamed vegetables. Then she found that she could cook them in a wok with olive oil and onions, which added a wonderful new flavor for him that he loved. She was able to nurse him back to complete health. This conversation changed my life for the next years to come. She didn't know it, but I started the same regimen she had utilized with her son. I began steaming zucchini which was the only thing I was able to eat for quite a while, but, over time, I added more green vegetables. Eventually, I began cooking in the wok and added more vegetables to the meal. My body healed one cell at a time over the next three years, and we still enjoy this meal frequently.

When I left the warehouse, the conversation I had had with this woman kept rolling around in my head, and I knew I had to talk with her again. I called the warehouse and asked if there was any possibility of speaking to the woman whom I didn't have a name for, but could described her appearance. I was told she was the manager and that she didn't call people personally. I pleaded with the person on the phone and said that the conversation with her at the warehouse had really affected me, and I would very much appreciate speaking with her just one more time. I left my number and hoped she would return my call.

She did call me back and gave me the single most important piece of information that would change my life forever—the name of the doctor that aided me in true healing. I had to plead with her to share the information with me. I reminded her how sick I'd been and that she had knowledge that could save my life. I was still not eating any solid food at that time and didn't know when that would be able to start for me. She couldn't recommend anyone but gave me a name. Somehow I knew that I had outgrown what the naturopathic doctor could do for me even though he was the beginning of this journey for health and complete healing. The new information came to me at the perfect time as did everything else that was related to my healing. God was giving me what I needed one step at a time.

The MD

I called the new doctor whom I now had the name for and made an appointment to see him as soon as I could get on his schedule. He was an MD but treated both traditionally and naturally depending on the needs of the patient. I needed the natural path to healing because I was allergic to all of the medications that had been previously prescribed. There were many prescriptions that sat in my cupboard untaken after just one or two pills were ingested because of the allergic reaction I experienced with the first or second dose. There was a reason for this as well. The perfect journey for me lay ahead.

I went to the first appointment with this new doctor, and there were, again, so many questions and a long questionnaire to fill out. The appointment took at least an hour. He continued to prescribe the liquid meal replacement and a number of other natural supplements, which could be purchased in the small apothecary in his office. I would see the doctor almost weekly for many months that lead to years, and eventually taper off over time. Sometimes I had a couple appointments a week when the pain was seemingly intolerable. I just needed the reassurance that I was doing everything I could and that my body would heal. The added supplements he prescribed increased our monthly medical expenses, but I knew that this would be my answer for my healing. We spent approximately $1,000 a month on the liquid meal replacement and the supplements I was taking. My body eventually healed cell by cell over the next three years.

Conclusive Diagnosis and Symptoms

There were many difficult times during those three years. I experienced so many symptoms that were scary and had to be dealt with day by day. Over time I asked the doctor about the blood work that was taken so frequently in order to monitor all my conditions. At the first onset of illness, it is natural to want to put a name to a disease. It somehow makes it easier for us to identify ourselves with a *name* that would then tend to identify who we are for the rest of our lives. After days and months that led to years of severe health issues, I asked the doctor if he had ever discovered what the name of my disease was called. He said that the cells from the blood tests had come back fluorescent which meant that it was conclusively lupus.

I was also diagnosed with fibromyalgia, which he said was a good thing; however, it didn't sound great to me to have to battle two illnesses. But the two disorders paired together meant that I probably wouldn't have the type of lupus that would be life-threatening. But it would mean that I'd feel horrible most every day with these diseases. He wasn't wrong. I couldn't imagine feeling any worse than I had been feeling. It was like having the flu day after day with no hope of recovering from it. Even so, my mind never did wrap around the possibility that I would live like this forever. I fought and fought to get well and kept that goal in mind with everything that I did over the three years I battled these illnesses.

There were times I wasn't sure that continuing to live in constant pain was worth living. Even though I didn't see myself as being sick for the rest of my life, the day after day struggle became overwhelming. There were days I had wished that lupus was terminal. Would there be a day that I would find relief and leave this world? Pain tormented every part of my body, and severe fatigue plagued me every moment of every day. I remember waking up one morning completely overcome with fatigue and thinking, *I wonder if I should actually get up and go to the bathroom or if it would be okay to just wet the bed.* I eventually gave in to better judgment because it would have been too difficult to clean up the mess, so I headed to the bathroom. But the fatigue, muscle pain, headaches, and stomach distress were constant in my everyday life. It was always there to accompany me into the day and end the day as well. In my waking, I would only look forward to the moment I could climb back into bed when the day was over. It was a grim existence at best.

I felt constant fear associated with being as ill as I was. I often wondered if I would wake up in the morning. Many nights I went to bed so sick that I thought it was a real possibility I wouldn't. Much to my surprise, each morning would appear, and I would dread taking on one more day. I was also frightened when new symptoms appeared. How would we deal with this one? Are there more to come? Dreading the dread was a pretty normal feeling during this time. In fact, there wasn't much I didn't dread. There were just different levels of it, and always an accompanying fear.

Unconventional Methods

This is definitely an uncomfortable topic, but I'm sharing this piece of my health journey because it may help someone. The only partial relief I experienced from the severe abdominal pain I experienced was doing enemas. I continued to keep in mind that a nurse at the naturopathic office had told me that it was safe to do them for a period of three years. I saw a gastroenterologist at the beginning of the illness journey I was on but was unable to get any relief even after all the testing that was done. I saw him one last time on a very unsettling occasion about two years into my work with the MD. The gastroenterologist warned me about doing enemas and told me that if I kept doing them that I'd more than likely end up with a colostomy, a bag attached to my body, and significant pain for the rest of my life. His words really terrified me at that time, and I had a significant emotional struggle about that doctor's visit. But I truly felt that I was being guided on every step of this journey and so settled my mind to continue with what I believed God was ordaining for healing. At the three-year mark, I felt a total lifting from needing to continue with enemas, and I stopped. I have never, again, had the need to perform one more enema.

Leaky Gut Syndrome

During the healing process, I was diagnosed with leaky gut syndrome. This is a situation where the bad bacteria in the gut had outgrown the good bacteria, and they literally ate tiny pinholes throughout my intestinal tract. This caused a whole host of symptoms like bloating, gas, cramps, food sensitivities, aches, pains, headaches, fatigue, etc. In order to alleviate this condition, I took a lot of probiotics. Typically people have to give up sugar and starchy foods that break down into sugar so that the yeast have nothing to eat and grow on. I had already given up sugars and carbohydrates, so the food issue was nonexistent for me. My intestinal tract eventually healed because of the food I was eating and supplements I was taking. Within the few years that I was aggressively doctoring, I took high doses of probiotics, but this was essential to my overall healing. I still take them today.

Fatigue

The kind of fatigue that is experienced with autoimmune issues is almost indescribable. The only similar type of fatigue I have experienced that comes close to the kind of fatigue I experienced during those difficult years is the kind of tired one feels after moving the last box out of an old home into a new home. The sheer exhaustion of a move comes close to explaining the severity of the fatigue that accompanies an autoimmune disease. The only problem is that this fatigue goes on day after day after day. Even after a full night's sleep I would wake and be just as tired. And much of the time, sleep was interrupted with some type of pain somewhere, but not necessarily the pain I went to bed experiencing. Fatigue, alone, was one symptom that caused an enormous amount of discouragement. These days, people drink high doses of caffeine with double and triple shots and down energy drinks like they are cans of soda just to stay awake. The feeling of constant fatigue is something we don't want to experience, but it was certainly an "every moment of the day" feeling for me at that time.

Pain

I never knew what part of my body would be in pain from one day to the next. It seemed that each day brought on a new set of symptoms until those symptoms started recurring again and again in a certain cycle that couldn't be predicted but would be sure to come. After some time, I began to recognize the symptoms as they circled back around. I found an article about lupus that stated that most symptoms once experienced would recur, but new ones wouldn't necessarily show up once the disease was well established. While others may experience kidney malfunction, I would not. Others may experience lung or heart problems. I would not. Still others would be hospitalized for other severe symptoms, yet I would not. I was thankful that the symptoms I had were mine and felt very fortunate to not be hospitalized for lung, heart, or kidney problems.

Fear

I was often afraid of the pain and afraid of the next painful moment that was sure to come. Nothing was certain except that pain would occur. During my daily driving around the city I would keep a constant lookout for the next hospital sign in case I needed to be seen in the event of an emergency. Most days were fairly normal, and I didn't need extraordinary medical care; although, it was always a worry. A typical trip around the city was fearful for me. I was always hoping that I would make it from point A to point B without an interruption due to some new symptom or problem. Since I traveled into the city every weekday for work, I knew where the hospitals were on my daily travels, but traveling to new places was always fearful for me.

I also never knew when some new health issue was going to pop up and deter the plans for the day. One morning as I was driving to work, I started having trouble breathing, and the skin on my neck and chest started getting red. I had put on jewelry as usual, but today and all future days, my body wouldn't tolerate the gold-plated metal. I quickly took off the jewelry during my commute in on the highway, and my breathing went back to its normal rate, and my skin turned back to its normal color. I wasn't able to wear jewelry after that incident for years and don't know why, and probably never will. I even had to let my pierced ears close up because my ears wouldn't tolerate earrings for many years. To this day, I wear very little jewelry. I may choose a strand of pearls or a simple chain, but it is very simple and usually hypoallergenic.

Scents

I became very sensitive to scented anything and everything. I couldn't wear perfume, and still don't. I'm not sure why strong perfumes gave me headaches and nausea and made me very light-headed, but they did. Even years later, I am sensitive to chemically produced scents. Most nature-based scents are lovely and are tolerated and healing to me, but I cannot be around the chemically produced scents that are often found in room deodorizers, perfumes, household products, personal care products, cosmetics, etc.

Light

I also became extremely sensitive to both natural and artificial light. I rarely turned on the lights at home, and only dim lights in the evening were tolerable. Sitting in front of my computer at work and under the florescent lighting at work also brought on the feeling of being under water and severe fatigue. There was no relief until I went home and could get away from the lighting in the workplace, but by then, I was suffering from severe exhaustion again. I have since learned that florescent lighting and the computer both give off something that can bring on lupus flare-ups. I requested filters for the lights above my desk at work that would filter out the ultraviolet rays. These were provided, but I was still surrounded by the UV rays from all the other lighting in the workplace.

I was also very sensitive to the sun. I couldn't spend any time in the sun, or I would get an immediate migraine, feel extremely weak, and feel faint. If the sun did touch my skin, it would leave deep red marks for some time after exposure. I wore large-brimmed hats and was fully clothed as much as possible during those days. Summer days were the worst, and it was difficult to be outside for any length of time whatsoever. I worked downtown at the time, and the short walk from the parking lot to the office was a difficult endeavor. I would eventually recover from these symptoms and enjoy many wonderful years in the sun, but at that time, my world became very small because I couldn't be outdoors for any length of time.

Comfortable

As most people with a significant illness feel, I was most comfortable at home. Other places caused discomfort in some way. Maybe the lighting would bother me or sounds or smells or other sensory issues would bring on a level of uncomfortableness that I didn't experience at home. Therefore, I didn't often want to leave our home to do much of anything. Of course, this leaves one feeling very isolated and can lead to not only a solitary life but low moods. I was trying to process this illness and all the pain that went along with it. It was easiest to do this in the comfort of my own home. One added comfort I had at that time was the constant closeness I had with God. He became my solace and my strength. I knew He was leading me every step of the journey, and I leaned on Him for everything. His presence during these years changed my life forever.

Body Changes

So many changes happened to my body over the three-year period. The pain was always there, but there were other changes as well. I had lost an enormous amount of weight. I weighed 105 pounds at my lowest, which I had weighed when I was thirteen years old. My weight would remain under 110 pounds for quite some time. My body literally looked like a child's body. At that time, I made a pact to myself that I would never complain about being overweight, if I should find myself in that place in the future. The struggle to keep weight on was so enormous that I would welcome the opposite struggle. Neither being too small or large is optimal, but when my life hung in limbo, I felt so helpless to change the circumstance I was in as my body was being bombarded with this disease.

What Is Lupus?

Many people have asked what lupus is because they have heard of it but don't really know what it is. The best explanation I can offer is that it is a condition where the immune system turns on itself. The body begins making an overabundance of antibodies. In a normal person there are 40 to 80 antibodies in one part of blood. In my blood, there were 640 antibodies in one part of blood. The antibodies can no longer determine what the foreign object they should be fighting against is, so they start fighting one's own body. This is experienced by tremendous fatigue, aches, and pains like the flu, headaches, and mimics of many other diseases. I experienced the symptoms of Sjogren's syndrome and Raynaud's syndrome just to name a couple. As long as it was the syndrome and wasn't the actual disease, it wasn't life-threatening. However, the symptoms were real and experienced just as if I had the disease. So my eyes and mouth were always dry, and my hands and feet were always cold and discolored. And rashes and skin conditions were abundant.

There were times that I saw my doctor two times a week when the pain became severe. Looking back at those days, I think there wasn't really much he did except listen to me and tell me to continue what I was doing. We did do some additional testing for stomach issues and found that I was dealing with a parasite called *Blastocystis hominis*. The test was less than comfortable. I sent away for a test kit and received everything I needed to complete the test at home. Part of the test was drinking a concoction that would completely rid my intestinal tract of any and all fecal matter. The word *uncomfortable* does not describe this experience; however, it didn't last forever. The parasite discovered wouldn't have even been detected by a healthy individual, but because of the autoimmune disease I was experiencing, I had significant issues with abdominal pain. It took nearly the entire three years to rid my body of this remarkably difficult-to-lose parasite.

I was also tested regularly for kidney problems during these years because lupus can be known to attack the kidneys. This test meant staying home from work because I had to collect every drop of urine output for twenty-four hours. Differing perspectives arise when these kinds of tests were being done. After completing them, I found it was simply a luxury to just be able to use the toilet as usual after twenty-four hours of catching every specimen. And I became very aware of and extremely thankful for running water and indoor plumbing. This was just a side benefit from the uncomfortableness that these random tests brought forth.

Food

For years, I prepared all my meals in a *wok*. I literally ate vegetables two or three meals a day and the liquid meal the other two or three times a day. I started out with green and almost transparent vegetables when cooked such as zucchini and cabbage. Then I began to sauté onions in olive oil and eventually added more vegetables. One by one, I added broccoli, carrots, purple cabbage, and then other squashes. Sometime down the road, I found I could add rice noodles. These were the first carbohydrates I had tasted in forever! It was heaven. As time went on, there was a brief period where I baked chicken and salmon. And then I heard from God.

A Deal With God

The healing that occurred over this journey was a combination of physical and spiritual. Each step I took was divinely guided. There are so many instances that I cannot write about each one. But I will share some throughout my story.

One evening after I had completed the evening enema, I was in the bathroom, and for the first and only time in my life, I heard the audible voice of God. As you can imagine, there were many times during my illness where I felt I lay in the delicate balance somewhere between life and death. God is closest to us during these times. The veil is lifted, and we are held by Him. I was down to my lowest weight of 105 pounds. I looked pretty emaciated. My grandparents had even come to live with us for a time because they were concerned that I may not survive.

I had just started adding chicken and salmon to my menu, and I heard God say, "Everything you need to eat is grown from the ground." I was thinking, *Are you kidding?* I had lost so much weight and really didn't know where this illness was going to eventually take me. So, I made a deal with God. I replied back, "Okay, I will eat no more chicken or salmon for a week, and if I've lost any more weight, I'll go back to eating them both." I weighed myself after the week, and I had gained two pounds. I heeded the words I heard from God and stuck with the deal. I remained a vegetarian for about ten years.

Shopping

I shopped at a national grocery store chain that had mostly organic fruits and vegetables. I would make the thirty- to forty-five-minute trip a couple times a week and then come home and prepare them for cooking. I spent time almost every day cooking them in the *wok* and making a little extra for the next day's breakfast and lunch. My doctor recommended that I soak them in a very weak bleach solution to kill any bugs since I bought organic and then soak them in distilled water for the final rinse. This process took so much time and energy, both of which were very precious to me. The trip alone was exhausting. After a couple of years, the same grocery chain built another store just ten minutes down the road from me. I remember crying with relief when the store was actually done. All the trips I had made to another city in order to purchase what I needed would come to an end. I would save time, and this meant more time for resting.

Travel

We took a couple of trips out of town during these few years, which required advance preparation as far as the food we would bring. One of the trips we took was to Myrtle Beach, South Carolina. We brought all the fresh vegetables with us as well as a hot plate and large pan so that I could prepare all my food in the room. It made for a really interesting-smelling hotel room even with the windows wide open.

Another trip we made was to our beloved Hawaii. We didn't want to have to prepare all our meals this time, so we brought pre-cooked meals with us to last the whole length of the trip. We weren't sure that we would be allowed to take the cooler of food with us so were prepared to fly right back home if we were denied upon arriving in Hawaii.

This trip gave me cause for great concern. I knew that I could survive on the liquid meal replacement long enough to get back home, but leaving the mainland when I was pretty sick was very unnerving. I wasn't sure what would happen to my body if I were to be in the sun for any length of time. Typically, lupus flares up with any sun exposure, and so I was pretty frightened by the thought of being on beaches and around the pool. I also wasn't sure that I could obtain the kind of medical help I would need if I experienced a flare, which could be worse than I had experienced in the past. I was, again, on the lookout for the next hospital sign everywhere we went. I needed to know where the closest medical facility was positioned at all times whether locally or during travel.

The first hurdle on our trip was passed as we were allowed to take all the food we had prepared onto the island. We were ecstatic! The rooms had microwaves in them, and though I knew most of the nutrition would be zapped out when I used it, there was also a calm that I could at least eat the food I was accustomed to eating and we could enjoy our time in our little piece of heaven on earth. There was still some fear and stress associated with our trip, but we vacationed without incident.

Surgeries

I had two surgeries during this time of health crisis. The first one was to take out a cyst on my right ovary. The doctor had kept an eye on it for some time and had elected to take it out surgically since it wasn't responding to any other methods of shrinking it. Prior to the operation, I was given a medicine that was supposed to help it to burst on its own, and it would have been taken care of within my own body. However, the cyst never burst, and the doctor decided it was time to remove it.

I had had surgery as a child but not as an adult and was concerned about all the medications I would need since I now had allergies to so many things. But we decided it was best to have the surgery done. We were hopeful that it would alleviate some of the intestinal pain I was still suffering from, but sadly it did not. When the surgery was over, the doctor said that the cyst was as large as a grapefruit and was, in fact, not the type that would have burst on its own. It was definitely a good decision to have had the surgery done, and I was thankful that it was completed without further medical incident.

My parents came to stay with us when the surgery was scheduled to help during the recovery. It was a blessing to have them help care for me and be close when I really needed their support. As I was healing, the abdominal pain I had been experiencing for the last two years became worse, and I asked the doctor about the surgery she had performed. She had done it through a laparoscopy procedure, so they had made small incisions and then inflated my stomach with air (gas) in order to complete the procedure. It was then that I truly recognized that the abdominal pain I had been feeling for so long was related to excessive gas in my stomach likely produced by the parasite, *Blastocystis hominus*. The sensations were both the same in feeling and severity. So, although the surgery didn't help my stomach issues, I felt that I had at least identified what could be causing the daily pain I was experiencing.

Before this first surgery, I had told the doctor that she would more than likely find endometriosis, so I asked her to please laser it off when she was doing the procedure for the cyst. After the surgery, she told me that she did find the endometriosis and had used a laser to burn it off, which would temporarily help with the symptoms. She also advised that it would probably grow back at some point and become painful for me, so we may need to perform surgery again in the future.

A little more than a year later, the pain of endometriosis had reoccurred worse than before. And when it became difficult to even sit at work due to the pain, I contacted the doctor, and we, again, went into surgery. Before the surgery, I had told her that my right side had often hurt, so if she saw that my appendix needed to come out to please do that as well. At this time, I was asymptomatic with lupus. However, we did experience an issue right before the operation. The anesthesiologist had brought me back and was getting me ready for the operation. He was talking to the other staff just like conversations in the workplace go when I started having a spinning sensation. I asked him if he had started any medications yet, and he said he had started the pain-relieving medications in a drip. My heart rate started racing, and everything started swirling around me. I could hear the heart rate monitor go faster and faster.

The next thing I remember was waking up in recovery after the operation in excruciating pain. Obviously, the anesthesiologist reduced the pain medication because of the reaction I was having, and all I could do was lay there breathing and wait until some of the pain subsided enough so that I could move. Quite a bit later, the anesthesiologist stopped by to see me, and I could see by the look in his eyes that things didn't go well. He wanted to make sure I was okay. I still sometimes wonder what happened to me, and won't ever really know for sure, but would like to have been a fly on the wall watching. As time in recovery passed, nurses came to check on me, and I asked for only acetaminophen. They complied with my request, and we waited until I could move. At one point, the wait was getting so long that my husband sent a nurse back to see ask me why I wasn't ready to leave. I explained to her that I was in too much pain to move to a wheelchair and get in the car to go home. So, we waited.

Eventually, I felt able to tackle the car ride home, and we made it straight home and into bed. The doctor had done both the endometrial scraping and taken my enlarged appendix out. The pain of those two cutting and scraping procedures was intense throughout the night. However, it is amazing how quickly our bodies adapt to pain and then work to heal so that the pain is lessened. By morning, the pain was tolerable with acetaminophen, and within a few days, I was handling the pain fairly well. As with any surgery I tired more easily, so I spent time resting as much as possible.

At the follow-up surgical appointment, I was given a clean bill of health. I asked the doctor how long the endometriosis procedure would keep me pain-free as well as fertile if we decided that children would be a part of our future. She said that the next six months were best for fertility, but conception was possible within the first year. After a year, the procedure would have to be repeated.

Twelve Months Later

Twelve months later, I felt the pain of menstrual cramps starting and was so disappointed that I'd have to have yet another surgery. I wasn't sure how the next one would go given the problems I'd experienced with anesthesiology during the prior surgery. However, as the next couple days went by, I didn't experience any blood flow, which seemed extremely strange. A week or so later, I had an appointment set with my regular doctor because I thought I had an ear infection. We discovered I simply had too much wax in my ear, so the medical assistant pumped what seemed like a gallon of water in my ear to clear the canal. And while we were in the office, I asked if they could do a pregnancy test. We were informed that the test was positive! The cramping I had experienced was due to the embryo attaching to the uterus, not the normal menstrual cramps at all. God had ordained this little baby boy to be conceived in the last month that the doctor stated we could conceive. We were ecstatic! I was also thrilled that I wouldn't have to have the surgery redone.

Babies

During each pregnancy, my health got better and better. Although I was asymptomatic at the time of our first son's birth, my blood tests still indicated that the ANA levels were at 1:640. Two and a half years later, we had our second son, and during that pregnancy, the ANA numbers were cut in half. They were 1:320. And five months after this little one was born, I found that I was pregnant with our third, and last, son. During this pregnancy, my ANA numbers were completely normal.

Since lupus is such a hormonal disease, a lot of young women are diagnosed with lupus when they get pregnant. My pregnancies, however, continued to correct the disease entirely. When I look back at when my symptoms started, I recall that the various allergies I had developed to medicine and foods started happening just after I had started taking the birth control pill. This hormone had started a spiral of health issues that I had no idea would become a struggle for me later in life. Thankfully with a lot of care from great doctors, a lot of money spent on natural healing, supplements, and organic foods, my body healed completely.

Health After Lupus

So many changes and new freedoms were found with the healthy new life I was given. Everyday battles of pain and fatigue had disappeared. The changes were small at first and took time, but after three years, they were hugely noticeable. The simple tasks of cleaning our home and cooking meals were easy again. I continued on the vegetarian diet for years, so our menu didn't change all that much. However, the ease of preparing became so much more noticeable. I could stay awake at night and not have to nap from the minute I got home from work until bedtime. Activities increased, and I was able to work out with vigor again. We traveled when we had the time. I was also more productive at work. I am eternally grateful for the path of healing that I was led to be on as it was a complete healing that I experienced and not just masked by medications.

Eventually I was able to eat more and more of the kinds of foods I had been allergic to for so long. And within ten years, I was eating a whole spectrum of foods to include meat, dairy, and wheat. I had the normal fatigue that a mother of three kiddos ages three and under would have, but I was healthy and didn't return to doctors for any kind of medical advice or consultation for years. My close friends and family told me that I should keep having babies, but my age prohibited me. I was thirty-nine when we had our last child.

Reading

While I was ill, I read everything that I could on natural healing, particularly healing from cancer. I thought if I did everything that people who had healed from cancer did, I would likely heal as well. This was ultimately my story. I read where miraculous healing occurred when people juiced for ninety or more days, putting nothing in their bodies except for organic vegetables and fruits. So, I juiced for a while. I read a fairly radical book about people who had become fruitarians—eating only fruit—that their diseases or ailments disappeared. I couldn't eat much fruit during my healing process due to the leaky gut syndrome and rebuilding the good bacteria in my gut but was very much intrigued by the possibility. I started seeing food in a completely different way than most people viewed food. It could save my life and yet just as easily destroy it.

I also read where people were taking trips to Mexico and going through intense clinics to purge their systems and free themselves of cancer. There were options to heal that I didn't even know existed until I was on a quest to heal my life. Reading about other's healing was so inspirational to me because it offered me hope. As a thirty-year-old person, I couldn't conceive of the possibility of living like a sick person for the rest of my life. It just wasn't in my capacity to think about or accept. So, the quest continued, and as it did, my health was restored little by little and day by day. I distinctly remember the first day I could clean my house, which I had been unable to do for a couple years. It was monumental for me! Some days it felt like there was no progress. And other days, I could see and feel the progress as compared to months prior or years prior.

At the end of the three-year wellness journey I was on, I was listening to a modern-day health guru who said that every three years, each cell in our body is made new (with the exception of our brain cells). I looked at my husband and said that this was exactly what I had just done even though I didn't know the science behind it. Every cell in my body was being made new over the three-year period, and I had a brand-new body that was well functioning and would serve me for years to come.

Spiritual Healing

Along with the physical healing I was experiencing, God was healing me spiritually as well. I spent a lot of time reading, sitting quietly, and meditating on Him. I had been brought up in the church as my father was a pastor. My grandparents were pastors as well. I knew what it meant to love God and be saved by His Son, but my actions at that time weren't in line with how I grew up and what I knew to be true. My character needed fixing. My actions needed to change. And so, He worked on me and worked on me and worked on me. He changed the path I had set for myself, and I began to seek Him and His will for my life. He started changing my spirit and infusing me with His love and wisdom. He began a work in me that continues through this current day. God stopped me in my tracks when I thought I knew the way. I was going the wrong way, and He had other plans.

The Lord, in His infinite wisdom, guided me every step of my wellness journey. He changed my heart and led me back to Him. I relied on Him for every step of this journey. And I am so very thankful that He didn't leave me alone. He could have, but He didn't. His presence was ever surrounding me. I sought Him and His peace, and He was faithful in providing it to me.

One of the things that generally accompany significant illness or any illness is accompanying emotions. There were times I didn't feel like I was normal. I felt weak. I felt like I couldn't control my emotions and found myself breaking down and often crying. These emotions kept me close to God and at His feet continually relying on Him. I found I could do nothing apart from Him. He has brought me close and has shown me the power that resides only by leaning completely on Him.

Peaceful Home

We had the great fortune of purchasing a home during the healing years. So many people have told us that that particular home was so peaceful. It was a haven for healing; although, we had no idea that our home would provide the perfect atmosphere for healing at the time we bought it.

We were also fortunate to furnish it and decorate it like I sometimes imagine heaven might look like. Just before we moved into the house, there was a closeout sale in a furniture store in town, and the person in charge of all the floral arrangements, framed art, and every other decorating item was marking everything down to nearly nothing. We filled our cars with so many floral arrangements that we looked like we were headed to a wedding. Our new home would be filled with the beauty and serenity that would be much needed for my healing as the healing years passed.

Holy Spirit

One evening after I had finished one of the most powerful books I had read about heaven and all its wonder, I thought God was preparing me to go be with Him. I was home alone, and the room was quiet. When I put the book down on my chest, the air in the room began to move around like wind was blowing through the room, but the windows were shut. I could see the outline of angel's wings around the top of the walls and ceilings. I was paralyzed with fear, unable to move. I truly thought it was my time to leave this earth. The angels were flying in a circle around the ceiling. After the wind had settled and the room returned to normal, I remember saying out loud that either God was getting ready to take me home or that God had a special purpose for my life and He was doing something amazing at that moment.

I now understand that what I had experienced was the infilling of the Holy Spirit. God had slowed me down so that I could completely accept Him as the Designer of my life. I had to get quiet long enough to hear what God intended for my life. The chaos of this world cannot give us the answers for our life. It is in the quiet that I came closer to God, not in the noise and clamor of day-to-day life and chasing dreams.

Visualization

As I have previously mentioned, I didn't envision a future of continued pain and discomfort. However, there were a few things that I did envision and were significant in my healing. Our minds are so extremely powerful, and I began using mine in a way to assist in the healing process. I was unaware of the power of the mind at that time but have been educated on the topic in recent years. Since the mind is so powerful, it should not be ignored even where our health is concerned. I'm not sure how these visions came to me, but these few imaginings assisted my body in healing.

During the years I struggled with the parasite, I would close my eyes and imagine that there was a little video game going on in my stomach and intestinal tract. I would imagine that all the little characters had laser guns and were shooting the parasite dead. There was a war going on in my stomach, and I was fighting it in my mind. Together we would win this battle.

I also had a couple spiritual visions. I imagined Jesus standing over my bed in a white flowing robe with blackness surrounding Him except for He and His robe that was glistening white. His arms were wide open to me. I would pray and believe He was healing me from head to toe. The peace that surrounded me engulfed me, and I could feel His healing power throughout my body. He was there every time I needed to call upon that vision, which was often during those years. I still call upon Him when I need His healing power.

Another vision I would call upon was a vision of the healing, crystal *living waters* in heaven. I would close my eyes and envision these living waters running through the streams in heaven and down small waterfalls. Then I would imagine these living waters were flowing through my body. Again, I could feel these waters healing as they flowed through my body.

One last thing I did with my mind was learning to alleviate migraines. I had such severe headaches during these years. This visualization began because there was an instance when I was scheduled for a chiropractic appointment during a severe migraine. The chiropractor was getting ready to do an adjustment when he felt the back of my neck. He told me that on one side the blood flow was enormous, so he put an ice pack on that part of my neck and told me to imagine that the blood was flowing in the opposite direction. I began to imagine that my fingers and toes were getting warm and imagined the blood flow was heading quickly in the direction of my extremities. Within a few short moments, the pain from the migraine was less and less until it eventually was gone. I used this method on many occasions back then and still do on the very infrequent times that I might suffer from a headache.

These visions helped alter the chemistry of my body. They provided healing that no medications could provide. And other than the migraine technique, no one told me to imagine these things, but they did become a part of my daily health regimen that helped support the healing of my body. Pain would return, but as it did, I would call upon these visions and feel them as often as I could. I truly believe these played a huge role in the healing process.

One Last Vision

I saw one more vision. As the healing process was coming to an end, I closed my eyes, and I saw myself walking through the fire and onto a mossy rock that was wet with dew. This led to a beautiful landscape of green grasses, trees, rocks, and lovely gardens. God was showing me that I was coming out of the difficult times and into His place of peace and rest. This was my confirmation that I would be completely healed very soon.

The mind and the spirit have so much control over the body, and I used them as best I could with the knowledge I had. God led me every step of the way and gave me the visions I needed to dwell upon. His love for us is everlasting. And again, during times of extreme physical impairment, the veil is lifted. For me it was lifted enough for Him to show me His love and show me He was with me. I was so amazed and anxious to listen to Him and allow Him to lead me moment by moment. His grace and mercy were sufficient for each interminable day.

Most people fall into each day and then into the next day. We don't really live. I had an opportunity to experience every moment because each moment was filled with some type of pain or relief from it. The fullness of each day was immense, and this time in my life was an opportunity to experience each second. I felt so tired and yet so aware in those moments. The awareness I experienced is unlike the moments I live today. We take so much for granted and skim over the beauty before us and ease with which we move from moment to moment. I wouldn't change anything during those years but continue to be thankful for the small things in life and am extra grateful for the big things.

Life After Lupus

I am ever so grateful to have had the opportunity to live an amazing life after spending over one thousand days fighting for my health and my life. With constant reassurance from my doctor and our Almighty God, I moved forward every day, and cell by cell my body healed. There were many nonbelievers in my life, and I didn't share most of what I was doing with anyone outside of my immediate family.

The only person who fully took this journey with me completely was my husband. He saw the effects of all the initial doctors, the medications they prescribed, and referrals to even more physicians, which offered little hope. When I started seeing the doctor who helped restore my health, my husband watched me. As the years brought on continued healing, he joined me on the vegetarian adventure. I was thrilled to have a partner to dine with and eat the same meal as myself because I had been preparing one meal for him and another for me. He also saw improvements in his health as we took this journey.

After three years of healing, I was completely asymptomatic, and life started to become normal. I didn't have the need to continue seeing the doctor anymore, so I just quit scheduling appointments. However, I did drive to their office for the next two years and purchase the supplements I had been taking while under his care.

Pregnancies and Real Life

Five years had passed since the onset and healing of lupus occurred. I had been asymptomatic for two years when we had the great pleasure of welcoming our first son into this world on December 4th. Going to the hospital to have this little bundle of joy was definitely stressful for me since I hadn't been to medical facilities much at all for the past two years other than the obstetrician. I had seen enough of doctor's offices and had enough blood draws for a lifetime. This stay was to be filled with medical staff, needles, pain, a cold room, and nothing to eat besides a popsicle or two. These were all familiar experiences and feelings accompanied by waiting and seeing and seeing and waiting. Nurses were in and out of the room all day checking on me. More needles and doctors came to evaluate the progress. And then of course, the real pain started.

I wanted to birth this baby naturally, so I wasn't interested in taking pain medicine or having an epidural done. However, as each hour passed, I began considering the need for help. By evening, I asked for an oral pain medication, which was quickly administered, and by 10:00 p.m., I was asking for the epidural. The pain wasn't so much the issue because I had a high tolerance for that, but I was concerned that my body wouldn't be strong enough to withstand the pain for many more hours. It was the stamina that I wasn't so sure I had at that point. My strength was weaning, and I didn't want to have to go to some extraordinary lengths to bring this little one into the world. So, the doctor performed the epidural without incident, and I began to feel the relief almost instantly. Within the next few hours, we brought our first baby into the world.

What an event this was for us! When I had been sick for so long, the thought of children wasn't on our remotest radar. We had no idea that children would be possible for us. Our main goal was to keep me alive and heal. It was unthinkable at the time to desire to bring little ones into our lives to care for when we were caring for me full-time.

We brought our first son home on a cold snowy December day. As a new mother, I was afraid of bringing a newborn home in the snow, so we bundled him up and put blankets around and over him to keep him safe on our journey home. My parents, grandparents, and aunt and uncle were waiting at our home to greet us and our newborn. It was a picture perfect December night, and all was beautiful and lovely in our home that evening.

Although I came to love every aspect of being a mom to our three boys, the road ahead was somewhat terrifying to me because I was completely unprepared for motherhood. I had worked a high profile job at that time, so I stayed working as long as I could before going on maternity leave. Initially, our time frame would have given us a couple weeks until the due date, but the doctor wanted to take the baby early, so we improvised. We managed to get the nursery ready and put up the crib just the night before we went into the hospital to bring our newborn son into this world. I hadn't had the luxury of reading baby or mommy books because the position I had at the time was all-consuming. There was no extra time or energy to read and learn all about what motherhood would bring. I really had no baby-caregiving skills at all. Fortunately, it was filled with so much love that any situation for which I was unprepared for was welcome, and I was determined to learn all that I needed to learn.

The Orange Drink

One interesting health incident occurred while I was pregnant. Every pregnant woman has to take a test to check for the possibility of gestational diabetes. I had the appointment and went in to drink a horrible orange (at least that was my flavor) sugary drink to test for potential gestational diabetes. I failed the first test, so a nurse called wanting to schedule another test with more sugary drinks for most of the day. There is no food ingested by mom before or during this test, and the whole procedure screamed *no*. I had so much testing done in prior years that I really wasn't up for participating in this one especially when it meant I wouldn't feel well before (empty stomach meant nausea while I was pregnant), during the test while drinking sugar for hours, and for some time after the test while recovering from the sugary mess. I told the nurse that I wasn't going to schedule the test at that time. She said, "Well, you have to!" I don't think anyone had ever questioned her or told her that they wouldn't be taking the test. After some more discussion, I managed to end the call. Instead of their procedure, I purchased a diabetes test kit and kept copious blood sugar notes to share with the doctor at the next appointment. The doctor was completely satisfied that I was not at risk for gestational diabetes and so did not require the horrible sugar ingestion again. I had learned to take charge of my health and not just go along with standard procedures.

Babies Continued...

Our second son was born two and a half years later on June 25th, and we brought home another beautiful baby to join our family. His big brother adored him, and once again, this little baby boy stole our hearts. He had blond hair that would stand straight up and blow in the wind. His eyes were sparkling blue and still are today. He had a very easygoing and sweet personality and was the only one of our infants who would love to go to sleep alone in his crib at night.

When our second adorable baby boy was five months old, we found out we were going to have another child! And when we learned that he was to be a baby boy, I rejoiced. I already knew the drill, had the clothes, and had the toys. We had no idea the joy our children would bring us. If we had, we would have started much sooner and had a larger family. However, my health would not have allowed us to have children prior to the time when we began our family. I was so thankful to be feeling well and living the wonderful life of a healthy mother of two with one on the way.

We welcomed our third and last son not quite fourteen months after our second child on August 19th. As we brought him home to join our little tribe, I was, again, thankful that my body not only withstood another pregnancy but my blood tests were totally clear of lupus. I was, in fact, functioning better than ever. This next little bundle of joy had dark hair and dark eyes. He watched everything that was going on around him and learned very quickly because he was intent on keeping up with his older brothers as he grew. We were thrilled to have our little family grow as it did, and by the time I was thirty-nine, we had a three-year-old, a one-year-old, and a newborn.

Each and every day of those young years were precious to us. We would move a couple times to accommodate our growing family, and when they were five and younger, we moved to a neighborhood where we would spend most of their growing up years. As you can imagine, I was an extremely busy mom of these three young boys. Days were filled with sweet mornings; daily trips to the park, pool, or museums; afternoon naps; and playful evenings We were so fortunate to live in a pool community, and have many lovely memories of long summer days and birthdays poolside. I was also very fortunate to be healthy in every way, and there were many days that I was very aware of, and ever so thankful, that I could fully enjoy my children in the sun by the pool. It hadn't been long ago that I couldn't even tolerate a walk in the sun without bringing on a total lupus flare. Now that my health had completely returned, I didn't need to worry that lupus would keep me from enjoying these precious days in the sun or anywhere the days would take us. Most days we played until we dropped.

Homeschooling

As our boys grew older, we decided to school our kiddos from home. We had schooled at home for preschool, so the boys were familiar with the process, but I wasn't sure how to proceed with elementary school. Thankfully, we found the support of like-minded families as we embarked on our first year schooling at home.

Each year, we would prayerfully decide what method of schooling we would utilize. We've participated in online schools, cooperative schooling, and charter schools. The years of schooling at home were some of the best years we had as a family. We took advantage of many field trips to museums and the zoo during those years. And again I was thankful to have my health in order to keep up with these three growing young boys whom I am blessed to have them call me mom. We easily managed the school workload in the time allotted and still had plenty of playtime. It was a lot of work to school three young kiddos but also very rewarding. They have all accomplished so many wonderful things in their short lifetimes, and we couldn't be more proud of them.

Fifteen Years Later

Fifteen years after the initial health journey I went through, my health started to deteriorate. It happened so slowly that I didn't really recognize it was happening. I was out of breath a lot, but not like before when it was hard to breathe. I was just out of breath and breathing heavy most of the time.

My husband and I had started a fairly aggressive workout regimen, and while on the treadmill one day, my heart rate was over 180. I told him that it seemed high, and he just said it was probably reading incorrectly on the treadmill calculator. I had taken the rate with my pulse, but we didn't pay much attention to that small detail, and life went on as normal for a while. We were busy parents of a now ten-year-old, eleven-year-old, and thirteen-year-old, so we felt justified in feeling tired and worn out. However, the labored breathing continued.

One day while I was putting the dishes away in the dishwasher, my husband heard me sighing. He thought I was sighing because I was unhappy with something he did, so he said, "What did I do?" I told him that he didn't do anything wrong, but that I was just simply breathing. At that point, he told me I should really get it checked out because it really didn't seem normal. So, at some point, I called and made an appointment with my doctor to see if he could determine the cause of the labored breathing. This next appointment would become a second journey that I would need to take in order to restore my health.

I drove myself to the appointment so that my husband could stay home and be with our children because we didn't leave them home alone at this point. And as I sat in the waiting room, I remember the television being on and patients glancing at it now and then while I looked for something interesting to read during my wait to see the doctor. There were plenty of magazines, so I picked one up and began to be taken inside the stories that were written. After a time, I was called in to see the doctor. Although I hadn't been in but a handful of times over the last fifteen years, he had been a great doctor for my husband and me.

One of the first things that doctors do is listen to the heart rate. Mine was 120 at rest, and the more concerned he got, the higher it went. He told me that he thought I had a heart embolism and that he suspected that a blood clot had already gone through my heart and was in my lungs causing the rapid heart rate. Again, my heart rate went higher. I was pretty scared at that point because the words "blood clot" seemed dangerous at best. I had not dealt with anything like this in the past.

He went into the next room, and I heard him tell the nurse that it looked like I was having pulmonary problems. I also heard him tell her that he was going to send me to the hospital. My heart rate increased once more. He came back to the room and told me that he'd like me to go to the emergency room of the hospital of my choosing and that he'd call an ambulance if I'd like. He said that I'd probably had the condition for over a month and that likely I would be okay to drive. The only thing that could happen was possible fainting. I was pretty shaken at this point but wanted to drive myself as I had done so many times in the past. This seemed no different.

I left his office and called my husband to tell him that I'd be going to the hospital. I asked him to call my parents to take care of the kids as we didn't know what to expect and how long I'd be gone. He quickly called and made the arrangements and was soon on his way to meet me. The emergency room intake was quick, and I was in a bed in a cold room within moments. There were people in and out asking questions and taking blood samples. I also had a CT scan of my lungs to determine if there was indeed a blood clot. It wasn't too long before the diagnosis was made. It was simply Graves' disease. There was a malfunction of the thyroid. My thyroid went into hyperspeed and caused so many of the functions of the body to go faster including my heart rate—easily diagnosed but not so easily treated.

So much was explained so quickly on that hospital day that we were not exactly sure what we were dealing with. They gave me medications to correct and support my heart rate. Rapid heart rates can result in heart attacks or stroke, so I was to be watched very carefully. If the medications didn't work and the condition wasn't reversed, then the protocol is to either remove the thyroid surgically or kill the thyroid with a radioactive drink. Neither of these options was desirable to me at all. I didn't want to undergo surgery, and I certainly didn't want to drink the radioactive iodine. I wasn't sure what else it would kill in my body besides the thyroid, and the possibility of it killing me was real, given my allergies to foreign matter. I didn't want to be without a working thyroid in any case because I still had many allergies to medications and didn't want to have to rely on taking a thyroid supplement for the rest of my life not knowing if I could take it all.

I began to research this disease just like I had done in the past. I read that antibodies attack the thyroid, which then makes the thyroid go into hyperspeed. Antibodies attacking anything could only mean one thing to me. I immediately called the endocrinologist and asked her to do an additional test on the blood she had just taken. I asked her to test the ANA levels for lupus. She said that she could have the test run, but she wouldn't know how to read the test. I told her that it was okay if she couldn't read it because I could. So, the tests were run, and the waiting game commenced. Again, these tests still took some time to be analyzed and the results passed on to me. Much to my dismay, my ANA levels were back to their original level of 1:640.

Many years prior, I had read that lupus is typically a very hormonal disease, so I thought then I might have trouble as I entered premenopause and menopause. The time had crept up on me faster than I had expected. I didn't realize that I was getting older because we still had fairly young kids at home. But here we were with yet another health crisis to deal with. At this point, I was wildly aware of my heart rate, and I could hear it pounding all the time. I'm not sure if it was getting worse, or simply knowing about my condition made me more aware of what was happening. I couldn't sleep well because my heart was always racing. It was like being on a treadmill twenty-four hours a day, seven days a week. At a resting heart rate of 120 beats a minute, there was no relief. I couldn't breathe slower or enough to reduce the rapid beating. And as expected, I was allergic to the medication. But something unexpected was happening too.

Not knowing that my healing was just around the corner, I was completely forlorn. I couldn't imagine having to do all the things I had done in the past to be well. I simply couldn't imagine it. I made an appointment to go back to the same medical office and start talking to the doctors there. The doctor who had primarily aided in my healing was no longer working there, so I saw his equally knowledgeable colleague. The first conversation was free; however, the next intake would cost $300, and they no longer accepted insurance. All the care that I needed would be out of pocket for us. This could not have been more horrible news.

We could not afford the medical care because my husband was on furlough with the airlines. We had no income at the time. The last time we doctored there, it was $1,000 a month on supplements and liquid nutrition. So, this new journey to regain my health would have to be different because we had no ability to fund my health issues as we had done before.

We drove the long trip home, and I was absolutely devastated. I had absolutely no idea what we would do. This health crisis brought upon new challenges that I didn't have the last time because I was a mother now, and the needs of our children came first. There were also no finances to draw upon this go-around and certainly nothing besides caring for the mere daily necessities was possible. We lived day to day believing that our needs would be met. God always provided. Every day and every month we were provided a financial miracle. We lived on miracles. We were protected except for this—except for me.

The night we saw the physician that we couldn't afford, I went to bed and prayed. I prayed that God would bring the healing to me as if I needed to remind God we had no way of getting it for ourselves. It was overwhelming, but God had a plan. I just didn't know what the plan was yet.

As discouragement and sadness came barreling into my heart and soul, I wrote a song. These lyrics are still so meaningful to me today.

> Don't make me talk
> I want to listen.
> Don't make me smile
> My heart is breaking.
> Just let me sit
> Be in Your presence.
> Help me imagine
> I'll make it through this day.
> Chorus:
> Lord, lift me up
> Beyond this struggle.
> Lord, lift me up
> Beyond this pain.
> Please lead me on
> Beyond what's seen, Lord.
> Help me walk into Your Mighty Plan.
> Lord, lift my eyes
> To see Your Glory.
> Lord, take my heart
> And make it Holy.
> Don't let me fall
> Far from Your presence.
> Help me walk through
> This pain in Victory.
> Chorus:
> Lord, lift me up
> Beyond this struggle.
> Lord, lift me up
> Beyond this pain.

Please lead me on
Beyond what's seen, Lord.
Help me walk into Your Mighty Plan.

(August 5, 2013)

The Answer

I had a niece whose husband transferred from Colorado to the northwestern part of the United States. They moved to where there was a private manufacturer that always kept families' needs first. They know the dangers of chemicals found in everyday items that families use regularly and made a determination to produce safer products to protect families. My niece started shopping with them because a friend recommended them for her daughter. Her two-year-old was suffering from severe asthma, and the chemicals that my niece was using in her home were exasperating her child's condition. So, she tried the store in her town and soon found that she loved everything she tried. People were friendly there, and she was meeting people who had gotten well from all kinds of different conditions. When she heard that I had been diagnosed with Graves' disease and the lupus had returned, she immediately gave me a call.

We were attending a family wedding when I got the call from my niece. She was telling me about this amazing store she'd found that had helped not only her daughter, but she had talked to a number of people who had gotten well from crazy stuff and recommended that I at least try the brand. I could hear the hope in her voice, but it was quickly drowned out by the festivities of the wedding. As sick as I was at this point, it took all my energy to simply be present where we were and then fly back home.

I spent many days and nights not getting any better. My heart rate was still very high. Of course, I was allergic to the thyroid medicine, so I had a full body rash, which lasted for some time because the medicine stayed in my system for weeks after stopping the doses.

The doctor's plan was to wait until the first medicine was out of my system before introducing a second medicine because we wouldn't be able to identify an allergy to the second if I was still reacting to the first. So, we waited.

In the meantime, my niece was persistent in trying to help me. I was really not interested in listening to her suggestions because I was somehow getting sicker every day. Once the diagnosis of Graves' disease had been given, I started exhibiting every symptom that the disease offered. And I didn't have any expectation that a simple shopping decision would affect my life the way my niece thought it would.

In the past, the organic vegetarian diet I utilized, in addition to the supplements I took, was the journey that I thought I would have to take again. However, we had no financial ability to entertain the possibility. I had gone to a local grocery store to try and mimic the same vitamins and supplements I had taken years before, but it was sporadic at best as we couldn't always afford them. They weren't doing my body much good anyway because of the quality of the vitamins and lack of absorbability percentage. It's really not the nutrition that is mentioned on the label that is important, but it's how absorbable the nutrients are that make an impact on the body.

Over time my niece's persistence and her endeavor to help me was successful. I started shopping with a manufacturer that made nonperishable consumable items much like we find at the local stores but without harsh chemicals and carcinogenic preservatives. In addition, they had discovered a technology that they utilized in their nutritional products, which delivered about ten times the mineral absorption than other brands provided. The reason I was able to make the brand switch was because the prices were about the same as what I was already purchasing, and in some cases less expensive. I primarily switched brands to keep my children safe as I was hoping to avert any possibility of them contracting something like what I had if at all possible. There was very little change in my health over the next couple weeks. However, after three weeks, my miracle came.

About three weeks later, I went to bed as sick as I had been but awoke the next morning with all my symptoms gone. It was crazy! The fog was lifted. All the flu symptoms that I had felt with the lupus returning were gone. The fatigue was gone. The heaviness was gone. The aches and pains were gone. The experience was almost unbelievable. It would be similar to needing glasses one day and the next morning waking up and seeing clearly. I remember it like it was yesterday. I kept thinking that this sensation may be temporary, and by nine in the morning, or early afternoon, or certainly by the evening, I would feel the heaviness of the disease once again. But that never happened. I never felt that way again.

I continued to see the endocrinologist for another nine months or so because she wanted to monitor my blood tests very carefully. Every month, the levels were less and less elevated. She never did prescribe the second medication to lower the thyroid levels. By the end of the ninth month, I received a letter from the doctor advising me not to come back because my blood levels were perfect. Another miracle had occurred. Once again, my health returned, but this time, I was well in three weeks instead of three years. God had a different path to heal that was far less invasive, lengthy, and costly. After going through the fire the first time, He showed me grace this second time. I have also seen others who have healed making simple changes in their homes and lives like these.

God had a plan to heal my body not just once but twice. Both were different plans, and both were miracles. There are still people who don't believe that healing from something like lupus, or other autoimmune disease, is possible. Because of my experience, I am not one of those people. I have been so fortunate as to see others get well too. We are all just people who kept looking for ways to heal and support our lives. I am thankful God guided me toward the right path at the right time.

Chemicals

My body is still sensitive to chemicals, but as long as I do the following, I am well:

1. Stay away from using harsh chemicals to clean my home.
2. Stay away from harsh chemicals, harsh preservatives, and hormone disruptors in my personal care products.
3. Stay away from preservatives, hormones, and other chemicals in my food.
4. Take highly absorbable vitamins and nutritional supplements that support my cellular and bodily functions.

Vegetarian Lifestyle

My most recent experience with food has led me back to eating the way I did when I was first diagnosed with lupus. I am, once again, a vegetarian. After a short time of making dietary changes, my energy improved, and my focus was clearer. I have not been ill with lupus again, but just changing my diet has improved my daily health.

After reverting back to a vegetarian diet, I also started losing weight. Over the last seven years, I have struggled with diets and lost a little bit of weight but always gained it back. I also struggled with fatigue. Twenty-five years ago, God told me that everything I needed to eat was grown out of the ground. I have been led back to this path and am convinced it should be the way I eat for the rest of my life. Some people balk at that, but all the reading and the research I have done over the years has lead me to believe that animal protein isn't necessary to live a vibrant life. In fact, some of the research I have done lends itself to suggest that less protein intake is better for a body that is prone to illness. It suggests that we need far less protein to sustain a healthy life. More information about what I am eating is outlined in a subsequent chapter.

A little sneak peek about my diet is my favorite morning drink. I blend vegetable protein with black coffee and oat milk. It is amazingly tasteful! I feel like the coffee shop made it especially for me, and yet, it is made in my own kitchen.

My health has improved beyond what I thought was possible at my age. I am very thankful for the journey I have been fortunate to take with God leading every step. His guidance and leading have been a blessing to me throughout my life. As soon as I am in need of the next step, He leads me there and provides. I am always seeking ways to feel better on this continued wellness journey, and I am constantly looking for more ways to stay healthy and become healthier every day.

As a result of feeling more energized, awake, and focused, I have been inspired to pursue exercise in a way that I hadn't been doing for the past seven years or so. And as I have given up the inflammatory foods, I have found that I can jog again. I haven't been able to jog for years due to knee pain, so I am very grateful to be able to participate in the well-loved sport! I have jogged most of my life, and it has been not only healing to the body but also healing for the mind. So, to be able to return to this form of exercise is wonderful for me. I am also seeking my personal bests as the regular workouts continue and can see the potential of extraordinary health as I move into one of the last chapters of my life.

Supplements

One of the key factors in my reacquiring my health the second time was finding as high a grade supplements and nutrition as I had access to twenty years ago but at a cost that was affordable. If you remember, during this second wellness journey, we didn't have any income because my husband was furloughed from his position with the airlines. So, our funds were extremely limited.

I was fortunate to have found access to the most highly absorbable nutrition on the market at a cost that was similar to what I was purchasing at the grocery store. I had attempted to duplicate the supplementation that I had received at the doctor's office years ago, but the grocery store brand simply did not have the solubility and absorbability that my body needed to be able to utilize the nutrition for wellness. I am so grateful that my niece didn't give up on me. She found the yes inside of my no. She knew she could help me, so she didn't stop connecting with me.

The supplements I take are:

> Multivitamins—Twice a day.
> Broad spectrum antioxidant—Twice a day.
> Omega's—And lots of them. Omega's are wonderful for the brain, joints, heart, natural inflammation reducer, natural mood booster, enhances clarity.
> Probiotics—I used to suffer with leaky gut syndrome, so probiotics are a must at least once, and sometimes twice a day.

Eye vitamin—My mother was diagnosed with macular degeneration, which is hereditary, so I supplement with a high quality eye vitamin.

Calcium and Magnesium—Twice daily.

DHEA—Twenty-five years ago, my doctor advised me to supplement with DHEA, and the research indicates that it is beneficial for lupus sufferers. I take a low dose of twenty-five milligrams twice a day.

Beneficial Household Changes

I didn't know that the things I was using in my home were filled with hormone disruptors. And since lupus is such a hormonal disorder, it was very important for me to eradicate those from my home. I learned that toothpaste, shampoo, laundry detergent, dish soap, and essentially anything with suds and bubbles contained an ingredient called sodium laurel sulfate. This ingredient is used in the production of many items we use in our homes. However, as I understand it, this ingredient turns into estrogen when it is absorbed into the skin which happens within thirty seconds of application. It was important for me to replace these types of items so that I wasn't exposed to further hormone disruption.

Another contributor to my poor health this second time around was the germ killer I was using to clean my home. I was kind of a germ freak. So, I was an avid proponent of bleach and ammonia. In fact, sometimes I used them together in the bathroom to ensure that I killed all the germs. This was extremely detrimental to my health. I also used the grocery store brands bathroom cleaners. Using these types of cleaners brought on a severe allergic response, and I generally had to follow up my cleaning with Benadryl. I had no idea that these products were so toxic to my body even though I had trouble breathing afterward. I really thought that they were the only way to adequately clean such messy areas. However, I now know that my beliefs about cleaning and killing germs were completely untrue. I simply cannot be around these types of products anymore. The dangerous cleaners have been removed from our home and are not welcome to return! In fact, when I am in situations where I travel and need to stay overnight in hotels, I even bring my own bedding because I am unwilling to put my health at risk.

I also learned that these products let off gases, which are terribly dangerous. When I first switched to a safe brand, I had intuitively boxed up everything I replaced and put the box in the garage. Later I learned that the off-gassing is almost as dangerous as using them.

Another chemical that we need not expose ourselves to is formaldehyde. This ingredient is known to be carcinogenic and should not be part of anything we use. Latest data indicates that cancer is just another autoimmune issue. Even if that isn't proven, my body was definitely affected by this ingredient. Again, I am glad I have found alternatives that are healthful, safe, and affordable for me and my family.

Lastly, poison control is contacted continuously at staggering numbers when children accidentally come in contact with toxic home products. I only wish I had had the knowledge I now have years ago because I would not have wanted any harm to come to my children because of my ignorance. In addition, it is quite possible I could have averted the second journey. However, there is a plan for everything. I am hoping that you will learn from my ignorance and avert any health issues or dangers to your family as I encountered.

There are many other manmade ingredients that my body does not handle well, so I stay as natural as I can. It is very important to be informed and utilize the information to stay healthy.

More on Foods

I don't eat meat anymore; however, if I did I would purchase organic because of the hormones injected into animals. I wouldn't want any added hormones introduced into my body that could possibly affect my health.

If I am unable to buy organic fruit, then I take the skin off before eating to reduce and eliminate the amount of pesticide ingested. Also, it's important to utilize a natural pesticide remover before peeling. There are various options available to help alleviate most of the pesticide issue and not expose our bodies to these unwanted chemicals.

Sample Meal Plans

Morning: Coffee, vegetable protein, oat milk blended

Snack: Fruit (I love grapefruit, peaches, nectarines, and bananas.)

Lunch: 2 eggs (either boiled or scrambled with onions sautéed in olive oil) served over a bed of rice.

Snack: Fruit

Supper: Vegetables (I enjoy sautéed onions in olive oil, add carrots, broccoli, yellow squash, green and purple cabbage.) served over rice or brown rice noodles.

Morning: Coffee and strawberry, banana, spinach, vegetable protein smoothie

Snack: Fruit

Lunch: 2 eggs and rice toast (no jelly).

Snack: Raw cashews with a banana and a teaspoon of pure maple syrup.

Supper: Broil vegetables and serve over rice or brown rice noodles.

Food I Avoid

Corn: I read an article years ago about a woman who had a severe corn allergy that replicated lupus symptoms. As soon as she took corn out of her diet, every symptom was alleviated. I wasn't entirely sure I had a sensitivity to corn until my young son asked me to hold his corn chips. Within minutes, my hand started to swell, and I had difficulty opening my hand back up. It was an easy way to tell that this inflammatory response was occurring inside my body as well. Corn is in so many foods, so reading labels is mandatory.

Wheat: I gave up wheat years ago for about five years. As time went on, I was able to add it back into my diet. However, I did give it up again a few years after reintroducing it at that time. As of late, I have given up wheat entirely. It had been causing my eyelids to swell, and I usually had to take Benadryl to counteract its affect. I feel much better having taken it out of my diet again and plan to maintain this restriction for the rest of my life.

Dairy: Dairy produces an inflammatory response in my body, so I have taken it out of my diet. I believe this is the reason I am able to jog again. Jogging was too painful for my knees and had been for a number of years. I truly thought I wouldn't be able to utilize this favorite exercise of mine. I am delighted to be able to run again!

Meat: I have taken meat out of my diet with no concern for adequate amounts of protein in my diet. I supplement with a high quality vegetable protein once a day. I don't notice any weakness at all. In fact, I feel much stronger and vibrant without it.

Soy: I am careful to not utilize much soy because it is another food that is a hormone disrupter. As my body ages and I experience more hormonal changes, it is important to not ingest food that will alter this natural process. It is also a fairly common allergy for most people, so I limit it.

Almond: I have an allergy to almond, so don't utilize the almond alternatives.

MSG: I stay away from all food containing MSG.

Grapes and Raisins: They tend to bring on lupus flares, so I do not eat them. I learned this when I had full-blown lupus. If I ingested them now, it would probably result in a headache.

Nightshades: Although I do not completely avoid nightshade vegetables, I consume them very sparingly. These include foods such as potatoes (sweet potatoes and yams not included; however, can affect estrogen levels, so I stay away from them as well), tomatoes, and peppers. Eating them regularly, or in large amounts, can bring on arthritic-type symptoms, bloating, etc.

Good news: I can eat rice and oats. I limit the amounts of both, but I enjoy them in moderation. There are a number of options available in local grocery stores that provide alternatives such as brown rice crackers, brown rice noodles, and rice bread (which I toast). I have found that these alternatives provide enough variety for me to eat without feeling deprived.

List of foods I regularly consume (as many organic choices as possible):

Fruit:
Bananas
Grapefruit
Raspberries
Strawberries
Black Berries
Peaches
Nectarines
Various melons on occasion

Vegetables:
Onions (usually sautéed in olive oil)
Carrots
Broccoli
Green and purple cabbage
Zucchini
Yellow squash
Spinach
Cauliflower (on occasion)

Grains:
Rice
Brown rice noodles
Oats

Spirituality

I would be remiss if I didn't mention the spiritual side of getting well. I believe we have a physical being that houses our spirit. We are physical beings that think and feel and are driven by an inward force. I believe in God Almighty, and I believe He guides my life. I continue to ask for His guidance and ask that He infuse in me His wisdom so that I may live the very best life that He has given me.

Our bodies manifest our inner beings. And when our spirit is not in alignment with His will, or we are seeking that which is different from His will, our bodies are negatively affected. That doesn't mean that if we are out of His will we will get sick. But my walk has shown me that my body is very representative of my inner being. My physical body becomes weak when I ignore my spirit. I try and take time every day to read the Bible, pray, and mediate on the Lord. In the quiet, He touches my spirit and body. In the quiet, He heals me.

Sometimes our pace in life is just too fast for our body to keep up. Our bodies are a great compass to lead us down this path of life. When my body gets out of whack, I check in with God and make sure there isn't a course correction to be made. I desperately desire to remain in His will.

Miraculous Events

God has led me every step of each of both of my health journeys.

The first doctor I was referred to had interned at a lupus clinic. He knew exactly what tests to order.

The liquid replacement meal that was prescribed by both the naturopath and medical doctor sustained my life.

The manager of the warehouse where I bought the liquid replacement meal led me to the medical doctor that would ultimately be the one with whom I would experience true healing.

The audible voice of God telling me to eat only things grown out of the ground was nothing short of miraculous.

The deal I made with God when I gave up chicken and salmon resulted in a two pound weight gain.

The infilling of the Holy Spirit completely changed me and the direction of my life.

My niece and her husband were transferred to the Midwest where she would find the solution to my next battle with lupus and Graves' disease.

Being led back to a plant based diet in these later years has resulted in reduced inflammation to further improve my health.

The quiet time I was fortunate to be able to take during both journeys has changed my heart, soul, mind, and body. I have never found God in the chaos. It simply isn't His nature. He comes to us in the sweet quiet. As I slowed down and sought Him, He became present to me. He has never left me, and I have learned to seek Him in my deepest need. As I seek Him, He provides answers.

Your Path

I wrote this book hoping to inspire those reading to keep searching for answers in their healing. If that is you, then may your path be revealed to you with God's speed. If the one who is ill is too sick to read and a family member is reading this, then please accept my encouragement to keep on seeking and searching for answers. There are ways to feel better and live healthier lives. If doctors and medicine has been your choice, there are also other things you can to do support a healthier life. It is my greatest desire to help others live a full and healthy life so that everyone can participate in life and do what they were meant to do.

If you or your loved one is sick and you would like to connect with me, I am more than happy to share more with you in the hopes that I can be of help to you. You may connect with me on various Life After Lupus social media sites, or by emailing me directly at andrea@andrealende.com.

If you are someone who schedules or oversees group activities, please contact me for a speaking engagement. I am available to speak to your organization offering various messages of hope, faith, overcoming trials, God's healing, natural healing, manifesting health and wellness, and more. Please connect with me at andrea@andrealende. com.

Stories of Healing

In some of the following pages you will read other people's stories about healing they have found. When I was sick, it helped me greatly to read about others who had struggled with their health and found ways to heal. Some healed with doctor's help, some naturally, and yet others healed utilizing a combination of both medical doctors and natural means. May your journey be one that leads you down a path of health and healing.

You may connect with me on various Life After Lupus social media sites, or by emailing me directly at andrea@andrealende.com.

I would love to share more with you with the hope of helping you and others on their wellness journey.

Rheumatoid Arthritis and
Hashimoto's Disease

"You know how much I love you, right?"

Brian just looked at me, his gray eyes dark with concern. He forced a smile and kissed the top of my head as I snuggled into his shoulder, shaking and nauseous. My heart felt like it was going to explode within my chest, beating faster, ever faster. I was lightheaded, and my mind was wondering if I was about to die. I hated hospitals, and this was my third trip to the emergency room within ten years. It was always the same, but this one was the worst; my heart was literally pounding me off my feet. Brian kept his arm around me, and we waited—an eternity, it seemed—to be called back into a room to have my vitals checked.

I mentioned that this was not my first time in the ER. A day in late May of 2007 had that honor. I had awoken that morning to a loud crash in the living room and realized that our two cats, Shaman and Chili, were having a bit of a brawl. Flinging myself out of bed while my now ex-husband, Mark, rubbed his sleepy eyes, I went in search of the kitties to calm things down. My heart beating from the excitement, I fed the little beasts and tried to calm myself down but found that no matter how I tried to regulate my breathing, I couldn't. I sank into a chair, lightheaded, and felt the world go into slow motion. A slow dialogue began in my mind with something larger than myself. It occurred to me that I was being given a chance to leave this earth, if that was what I had wanted to do. In what had to be seconds, but felt more like an hour, I weighed out my options in silence.

I was unhappy with my life, my marriage, my business, and my body. Four years prior, I had been diagnosed with rheumatoid arthritis, and little by little, everything that I had loved to do was falling from my grasp, quite literally. Once strong and energetic, I had been a massage therapist, a yoga enthusiast, a real estate rehabber, and someone who loved to explore the outdoors with daily walks and hikes. Now I was short on energy, and my hands struggled to work. My feet betrayed my will with pain when I walked. Even journaling was difficult, because holding a pen and writing down my thoughts only sent cramps throughout my hand and up into my arm. All I could do was sit in a chair and read with my cats by my side.

I realized that, in this particular moment, I was almost ready to go. Almost.

"Is it worth staying?" I asked to the silence. All I got back was the feeling that it was my choice. And with that, another feeling— regret, deep regret for what could have been, deep regret that I hadn't done anything of significance yet. I was only thirty-eight years old, and what if there was more? What if I still had a chance to do this life right?

"All right," I said to the silence. "But things need to change. If they change, I'm in."

Time sped up, and the lightheadedness was back in force. "Mark!" I called out as loud as I could manage. "I need to go to the hospital. Now!"

* * * * *

After two and a half days in the hospital, I was released with blood thinners and anti-anxiety meds. All the doctors could find, after almost nonstop tests and two overnight stays in what seemed like hell, was that I was anemic and had fibroids in my uterus. With the blood thinners, I was forbidden to eat leafy green vegetables due to their Vitamin K count, which I now know is critical for Vitamin D synthesis, something that most people dealing with autoimmune issues are short in. As a former massage therapist and current healthy lifestyle advocate, I hated this idea. Behind my husband's back, I threw out the meds, and I began to research on how to strengthen my body and blood.

Three years later, the difference in me was night and day. I had divorced my husband and had become a colon hydrotherapist; I was a champion of cleansing the colon and the liver, and I was all about supporting the digestive tract through fiber and nutrition. I learned about parasites and leaky gut, and my daily food came from a powdered meal replacement supplement. For sixteen months, I did not eat any solid food—nothing but canistered powder and water. I felt stronger and energized, but social engagements were tricky, as I found that most of my friends would gently ridicule me because of my choice to not eat "real food." I'm sure a few assumed that I had an eating disorder and watched me very closely. However, I was ready to try extreme measures to knit my digestive tract back together, and my weight, after a twenty-pound weight loss, stabilized and looked reasonably healthy.

Although I felt better, this didn't stop the RA from progressing. It slowed, but I still noticed small losses over time, and I knew that I hadn't cracked the answer yet. And then I had to deal with a job layoff that left me financially in trouble. My meal replacement, which cost me over $700 per month, had to be let go. I suddenly found myself back on solid food, and that led me to ER visit number two.

Within a week of my new diet, my face broke out with an acne rash worse than anything I had ever experienced as a teenager. My skin was inflamed with heavy cystic pimples that filled my forehead, chin, and cheeks. For three weeks, I struggled with acne products and cleansing routines. And then, the pounding heart began again. I was back in the ER, afraid again that I was having a heart attack. Of course, no one could find anything, except that I was still slightly anemic. Hours later, my EKG was normal, and I was free to go home. I still had no answers but was strangely comforted that my heart seemed to be okay. I was off to do more research on my strange condition.

Since I had been first diagnosed, I had studied nutrition, colon hydrotherapy, energy work (I was now a Reiki Master), and now I found a new job where I learned about subtle light and sound energy healing. This was my introduction to the autonomic nervous system (ANS) and trauma and how a dysregulation of the ANS is linked to autoimmune diseases. Modern western medicine views autoimmune issues as "the body attacking itself." However, I was learning that a chronic state of stress within the ANS creates an atmosphere of mixed signals within the body; the body can either be in fight or flight (sympathetic) or rest or digest (parasympathetic) mode. However, when forced to deal with chronic stress or trauma over a long-term period, the body is forced to survive under conditions that the mind perceives as "unsafe." This will trigger a confused messaging within the endocrine system while exhausting the adrenal glands, and then the thyroid gland is put into jeopardy. Everyone with thyroid issues (and autoimmune, in general) should check to see if they are in adrenal fatigue.

This brings me back to ER visit number three.

I was brought back to a room and given several blood tests. My EKG stabilized, but my doctor told me that my thyroid was barely functioning. I was diagnosed with Hashimoto's thyroiditis, which is an autoimmune disease of the thyroid. In hindsight, this probably should have been the original and correct diagnosis from years prior, but it had been missed time and time again. What brought everything to the brink this time, out of the blue? I was now finally, and fully, in menopause, and it would seem that every time my hormones changed, so did my thyroid.

Two and a half years on Armour Thyroid did nothing for my health, and my doctor kept wanting to increase my medication. My heart rate still beat between ninety to one hundred beats per minute; I was prone to anxiety attacks; I continued to have night sweats even though I was postmenopausal, which made my sleep patterns horrible; and my doctor was now ready to send me to a cardiologist despite my concerns that my heart pounding was a regulatory issue (thyroid and endocrine system), not a cardiology issue. I went home that day with a renewed determination, and further research was done.

First, I began slowly weaning myself off my thyroid meds, and I did this over a seven-month period. Second, I began taking adaptogenic herbs such as ashwagandha, holy basil, ginseng, maca—these herbs support the adrenal glands and take stress off the thyroid. I also took myself off caffeinated beverages, since those tax the adrenals even further. Next, I realized that my digestive tract was still problematic because, obviously, some nutrients were not being absorbed properly. I did research and found an amazing company that has nutrition with a proven track record of bioavailability and phenomenal laboratory results. I supplemented that with sublingual (held under the tongue) B12 and magnesium to ensure the absorption of those two critical elements. Also, from that same company, I found a high-quality fiber product that has prebiotics within its formula and also added probiotics to replenish my digestive tract. The company also had vitamin D and Omega 3s and 6s, which are critical for people dealing with autoimmune issues. To top that off, I added DHEA, something that anyone over thirty with autoimmune issues is usually short in, as well.

Between the supplements and weaning off the thyroid meds, I started to feel better. Seven months later, I stopped the thyroid medication and, a year later, have not looked back. My night sweats have stopped. My heart rate is almost normal, since at my last dental visit I had a pulse of seventy-six beats per minute. My panic attacks stopped, and I sleep well through the night. And I should add, my energy is back; I no longer need a nap or two throughout the day.

I think back to that day when I had my silent conversation, the one where I chose to live. I think back to the regret I felt at not having made a difference. After over twenty years in alternative health and after dealing with autoimmune issues for at least the last sixteen years, I have tried so many different products and supplements, seen endless doctors and naturopaths, and struggled to find answers. My journey has given me knowledge I could never have gotten from any other way but through experience and trial and error. I am so grateful that I have found a company that provides products that support the body in a nontoxic, bioavailable way. I feel so blessed that now I can help others through the darkness of autoimmune and help them to find a better way.

Never give up hope. There *is* life after autoimmune, and it can be a happy, healthy one!

Tracy

Diabetes Control

With my first child, I had gestational diabetes and was put on a strict diabetic diet for the remainder of my pregnancy. I was also told that this condition can put me at higher risk of becoming a diabetic as I age. Diabetes runs in my family, so I am at an even higher risk of high blood sugar. At one of my last physicals, my blood sugar was higher than normal, and I was told to be careful about my sugar intake. I found an online store that has exceptional nutritional products and started using a shake that was designed to reverse prediabetes. There are so many wonderful natural ingredients in it that help regulate blood sugar, and a year later, my blood sugar had returned to normal levels. I am always looking for natural remedies for health instead of taking prescription drugs, so I am very thankful for the technology I've found to help me remain healthy as I age. I've also found a fiber that helps my intestinal tract be healthy, which is so important for my overall health. Since our immune system is a huge part of what's in our gut, I have found I'm much healthier when I take fiber loaded with probiotics and prebiotics, vitamins, and herbs.

Ronna

Blood Pressure

My name is Scott Chadwick, and I recently made a change in my daily life that has turned out to make a big difference. As the father of two very active boys, I decided to step it up and try to be a good role model for them. I cherish my boys, and I want to be able to watch them grow and become men and maybe someday become fathers too.

I grew up like my boys, very active and into all kinds of sports. Fitness was important to me, and at a young age, it was effortless (boy I wish I could go back to those days). As a young man, I joined the navy where I continued to be active and never had a problem with my weight. My parents are also in good shape, but they were both diagnosed with high blood pressure in their thirties and forties and as a result were placed on high blood pressure medicine. In my thirties when my blood pressure started becoming borderline high, my doctor also put me on high blood pressure medicine.

In my late thirties, I had lots of bad lower back pain and a herniated disk when I turned forty. I underwent a spinal fusion surgery that was very hard to recover from. During this time, I was not active at all, and before I knew it, I was gaining a ton of weight. A couple of years ago, I recognized that I needed to do something about my weight gain because I had little to no energy and felt fatigued all the time. I was dependent on my blood pressure medicine to maintain a safe blood pressure, but I hated to go to the doctor for fear of what he would tell me about my health. I would go only when necessary to receive a renewed prescription of my medicine. I knew I needed exercise, but I did not have the energy to do so. On breaks at work, I would nap due to my exhaustion.

March of this year, I was taking my oldest son to a baseball game. We stopped at a fast-food place on the way there, and we both got breakfast sandwiches. While driving to the game, I began eating my sandwich, and I swallowed a big bite that got stuck in my throat. Pulling over to the side of the road, I was seeing stars. On the side of the road, I could hardly breathe, and I honestly thought I was going to die. I didn't, the food finally went down, and it was at that moment I decided to make a change in my life.

I began to force myself to take walks even when I would much rather sleep. I did not go on any crazy diet, but I watched my portion size much more closely. Everything in moderation. Also, around that time, I bought some items off a neighborhood Facebook marketplace where I met a now friend who turned me on to some nutritional supplements with real absorption. She told me about the difference these supplements made for her, and I could tell that she really believed in them. I was very skeptical, but I ended up giving them a try. I didn't notice a major change in the first couple months, and I almost quit altogether, but I ordered another month's supply anyway. Before the end of that third month, I began to feel like I had a little bit more energy.

I was starting to believe they were helping. Of course I continued to walk three to four days a week too. Two months ago, I visited my doctor, and he was impressed with my weight loss. I told him of my desire to eventually get off high blood pressure medicine, and after looking at my lab work, he said he thinks it is a real possibility. In March, I was weighing about 212 pounds at five feet, ten inches. Almost seven months later, I have lost more than thirty pounds, and most importantly, I feel better than I have in years. I will be forty-four in a couple months, and I feel like I did when I was thirty-four. I look forward to three- to four-mile walks every day with my dogs. I have been receiving compliments from people about my appearance, which has done wonders for my confidence. This morning when I stepped on the scale, I weighed 181.2 pounds, and I feel great.

There is hope of better health when giving your body the correct absorbable nutrition and making some simple changes. A few days of walking a week has also helped my transformation. These simple changes have greatly improved my life, and I am thankful that I continue to see improvements as I am consistent.

ADHD, Depression, Anxiety

I come from a family of ADHD, anxiety, and depression. My son has ADHD, and I have the other two. After trying many different things and lots of reading, researching, and talking to professionals, I found what worked for us. I removed all artificial color from our diets and switched *all* our cleaning and personal care products over to a brand that doesn't have harsh chemicals in them. I found what chemicals do to our body and why so many people were on this "go green, non-GMO, clean living" kick! It really does interact with our bodies in so many negative ways. God didn't create these things, and we are not only eating them, but smothering our bodies in them and breathing them. Although our family is not free from hereditary issues, they are very manageable. The difference in my child is so drastic that had I made the simple changes I made years ago, we may have never gotten the ADHD diagnosis.

Toni

Migraines

I was diagnosed with classic migraines years ago. I was having severe headaches that had started to affect my vision. On one of
the first occasions my vision was reduced to what seemed like I was
looking through a kaleidoscope with colors surrounding my field of
vision. My husband took me to urgent care to try and determine the
cause. I was referred to an ophthalmologist who diagnosed me with
classic migraines. The medicine, Relpax, was prescribed for me to
take at the onset of a migraine to minimize the symptoms. I would
keep it on hand at all times because if I accidentally ran out of it I
would find myself, again, in an urgent care facility in order to combat
the full migraine and vision problems. This was my norm for five and
a half years.

I made a simple change in my home and don't suffer from
migraine headaches any longer. About 10 years ago I was regularly
using bleach and other toxic household cleaners when I switched
to a brand that uses no toxic chemicals. I hadn't considered that
the chemicals in my home could be causing the migraines until I
switched brands and found that I was no longer having the headaches. This almost went unnoticed as well. My husband had asked
me if I had renewed my prescription for Relpax, and I said I hadn't,
but I also hadn't used it in over six months.

As time went on my health was maintained and I haven't ever
filled a prescription for Relpax again. I am very thankful that a simple
change in the brand of household products I purchase has had such
an amazing affect on my health because the medicine I was on was
very strong. I could literally feel it begin to work as there was always a

tingling sensation behind my ears. There are a number of side effects of most drugs and the one I was on was no exception. So, I am very grateful to no longer need to be taking Relpax. As a health enthusiast, I am always looking for ways to be naturally healthier and grateful to have found a non-toxic brand for my home and my family.

Dawn

Eczema

My name is Jovan and I am a wife and mother of four beautiful children. They range in ages from four to seventeen. The wellness journey for me and my family led me to go green as I was searching for help for my youngest child. She was born with so many problems that I wasn't sure where to start.

I had had a complicated pregnancy, and seeing her struggle so much as an infant left me feeling discouraged with our medical system in general. My daughter had struggled with feeding from the day she was born. I was nursing and had plenty of milk, but she wasn't eating enough for some reason. After we were discharged I was going in for daily visits with lactation nurses for ten days. We were back and forth with providers because of her inability to gain weight, but were not finding any answers. When she was two months old she required a feeding tube. At nine months old I was seeing an allergist because she was breaking out in horrible rashes all the time. She was diagnosed with numerous food and contact allergies as well as severe eczema. The allergies made her eczema flare ups extremely severe. She suffered from chronic skin infections which turned into MRSA. We were given every steroid cream available, but nothing helped. We were then prescribed seven months of phototherapy. During these seven months of phototherapy she had to stay out of the sun from 10am to 6pm, so we completely missed summer with her that year. It was miserable for the whole family.

One day I was at the library and picked up a book on toxins. After reading just a few pages I decided to look at the ingredients in my cleaning products to see what toxins I had in my house. I was in shock. I could not believe how many harmful chemicals and toxins were in my household cleaners. I was always cleaning to kill everything I could thinking I was doing the right thing for my family. However, I was doing more harm than good.

Once I learned about how harmful the chemicals were, I started making my own cleaning products, mostly with vinegar and essential oils. My husband HATED the smell of vinegar. But I had relief knowing that I was keeping my kids safe, and raising them in a toxin free home. Since then I have found a brand of household products, for both cleaning and personal care, that is toxin free. Our whole family loves the new fresh smells! I don't have to use any more vinegar, and I love the effectiveness of the new brand. They work better than the toxic ones I was buying in local grocery stores.

As I switched my home over, I was also thinking about the planet. Typically we use an extraordinary amount of plastic. The store I have found concentrates their products so they use far less plastic than what I was buying. I know I won't fix the entire planet's problem, but I want to at least lighten our carbon footprint.

My daughter's eczema started to clear up on mostly her limbs within 7 to 10 days of reducing the toxins in my home. And today as I write this, I can tell you she is doing 100% better. She is a bubbly and happy little girl.

Since I started my wellness and green journey, I have had 3 extended family members diagnosed with cancer. I am continually looking for ways to help keep my children healthy and safe. The research I have done suggests that cancer risks are lowered by reducing and/or eliminating toxins as much as possible. We will always be subjected to environmental toxins outside of our control, but I will continue to reduce the toxins in our home and in our food for the health and safety of my family as much as possible.

Jovan

About the Author

Andrea Lende is an inspiring and uplifting author who will instill gratefulness in your life's journey. In this amazing biography, she journals her experience from illness to health, sharing exactly what she did to get well. Her path through her course of sickness to newfound life has heightened her spiritual being. As such, she also writes daily prayers and meditations, as well as a book with excerpts detailing God's faithfulness during financial famine. Andrea's road from sickness to health is astounding and has had a life-changing impact for her and others. She speaks on the power of life's adventures that we are all challenged with and fortunate to overcome. This determines our new strength as we push our limits and then surpass them. Look for additional books to be published soon.

CPSIA information can be obtained
at www.ICGtesting.com
Printed in the USA
LVHW041158171120
671900LV00006B/540